CLINICIAN TO COACH

SECRETS TO BUILDING YOUR SUCCESSFUL HEALTH COACH PRACTICE

JESSICA DRUMMOND, DCN, CNS, PT, NBC-HWC

CONTENTS

Difference Press

Washington, DC, USA

Copyright © Jessica Drummond, 2020

All rights reserved. No part of this book may be reproduced in any form without permission in writing from the author. Reviewers may quote brief passages in reviews.

Published 2020

DISCLAIMER

No part of this publication may be reproduced or transmitted in any form or by any means, mechanical or electronic, including photocopying or recording, or by any information storage and retrieval system, or transmitted by email without permission in writing from the author.

Neither the author nor the publisher assumes any responsibility for errors, omissions, or contrary interpretations of the subject matter herein. Any perceived slight of any individual or organization is purely unintentional.

Throughout this book I have used examples from many of my clients' personal lives. However, to ensure privacy and confidentiality I have changed some of their names and some of the details of their experience. All of the personal examples of my own life have not been altered.

Brand and product names are trademarks or registered trademarks of their respective owners.

Cover Design: Jennifer Stimson

Editing: Erika Parsons

Author Photo Credit: Jenn Reid

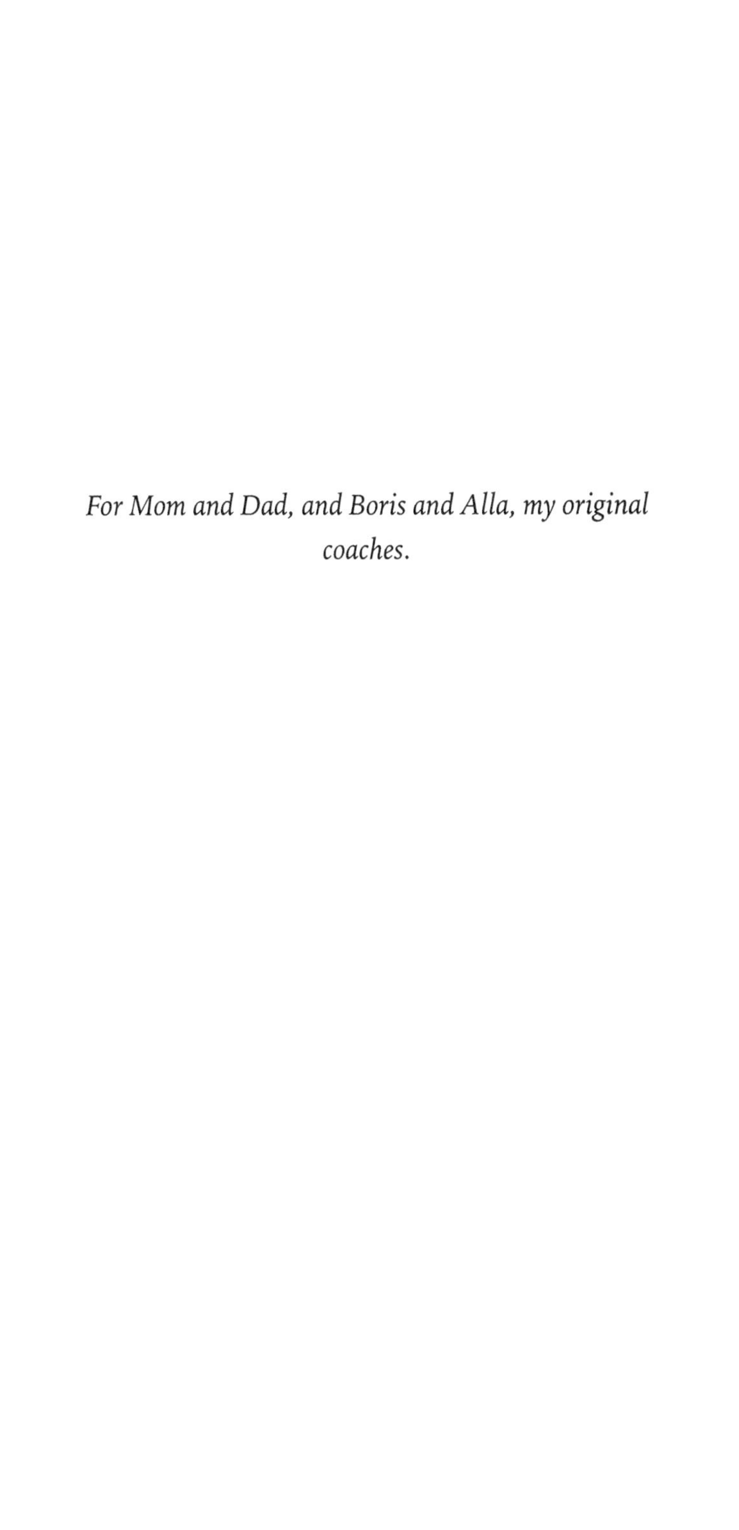

For Mom and Dad, and Boris and Alla, my original coaches.

1

THE TRANSFORMATION IN
HEALTHCARE IS HAPPENING NOW:
DON'T BE LEFT BEHIND

For my entire two-decade career in healthcare, the broken healthcare system has been functioning like a drug addict. It destroys the very healthcare professionals who come to it with good intentions of taking care of others. It's obsessed with money over people. It does a terrible job of promoting health. At best, it rescues people from the brink of acute disaster – but only for a fleeting moment. It doesn't address the root causes of the pain.

Now we know what will finally bring that system to its knees, what will finally allow it to feel rock bottom and know that it's time to do the work to heal itself so that it can mend the broken promises it made to every professional and patient that it has hurt.

As I sit here today, we are witnessing the global coronavirus pandemic. This pandemic is the bender that is finally bringing us to the brink of disaster.

As clinicians, we now have a choice. Transform or die.

The healthcare system must now be reinvented. Despite the years of pain and burnout you experienced at its hands, you now have the opportunity to be a part of the ushering in of the new paradigm. But first, you must take the opportunity to transform yourself and how you practice from the clinician mindset to the coaching mindset. No longer will you be the God who "fixes" your patient. You will have to let go of the ropes of control and learn to prioritize your own health, your own boundaries, and trust that the patient sitting in front of you has innate healing wisdom of her own.

To be successful in this new paradigm, you will need to learn and practice three new skill sets: coaching communications skills, nutrition and lifestyle medicine, and, perhaps surprisingly, the skills of marketing and sales. We'll get to all of that later. But, first let's talk about what this transformation looks like.

IS HEALTH COACHING REALLY LEGITIMATE?

The grand idea that transforming how we practice as clinicians from a clinical, top-down perspective, to a coaching partnership perspective, will revolutionize healthcare as we know it might seem overstated. One of the reasons you might be skeptical about the importance of this transformation is because health coaching has a questionable reputation right now because no one really knows what it is. "Health coaches" are popping up all over the place as Instagram influencers selling supplements and promoting diet and fitness fads. But, at its core, that's not what health coaching is. To be fair, health coaching does have a branding problem, because until very recently, it was not a clearly defined area of healthcare practice. And even now, there are a lot of gray areas in the scope of practice and no clear legal definition of the term "health coach."

The good news is that the professionalization of health coaching practice is happening rapidly. There is now an approval board for health coaching education programs that requires training programs to submit to a rigorous approval process and annual audits. The National Board for Health and Wellness Coaching has done an exceptional job of collaborating with many stakeholders to elevate and clarify health coaching practice. I appreciate their hard work, and what they have done to elevate our health coach certification program immensely.

Now, to be a practicing health coach at the highest level, you can take an international board exam similar to all of the clinical board exams that other health professionals like physical therapists, nutritionists, physicians, and nurses take. I strongly recommend that you commit yourself to this level of training and board certification if you want to be a leader in ushering in this new paradigm in healthcare.

I HAVE A CLINICAL LICENSE. CAN I BE A HEALTH COACH?

The most common question that holds clinicians back from transforming their practices to a coaching model, and the reason why so many health fad charlatans can thrive, is because we are afraid that somehow practicing health coaching will put our clinical license at risk. Nothing could be further from the truth. Legal professionals, like my own attorney, Lisa Fraley, have dedicated their practices to being sure that clinicians who want to use the coaching model to drive their practice forward can do so safely and effectively under the law. If Instagram influencers can legally educate the public about the benefits of powdered greens supplements, then certainly there is a way for you to much more effectively promote healthy lifestyle behavior changes for your patients.

WHAT IS HEALTH COACHING?

That begs the question, "What is health coaching?" Is health coaching all about teaching people how to eat, what supplements to take, and whether or not they should lift weights or run, or is it more than that?

At its core, health coaching is the perspective that the patient sitting in front of you comes to their appointment with you with wells of innate healing wisdom. Your patient likely also would benefit from improving their day-to-day foundational health behaviors as a path to long-term, root cause healing of most of the common conditions humans struggle with today. If your patient could learn to tap into her innate healing wisdom, step into her power, and fill in any gaps in her health wisdom by consulting a team of health professionals (including, but probably not limited to, you) and take daily steps to move, eat, sleep, and manage her stress better, she could heal even her most complex chronic health challenge instead of band-aid it with lists of medications or surgery after surgery.

Health coaching is not the best perspective for a very few health challenges such as acute injuries or accidents, or acute organ damage like a heart attack or stroke, though it could prevent many of these from ever occurring. But for everything else from chronic pain to cancer recovery, chronic fatigue to hormonal symptoms, health coaching is the perfect healing model. Often the day-to-day habit transformation that the patient does will be accompanied by medical or surgical intervention, but both will be far more effective if the foundations of health are put into place with a lifelong commitment to the coaching model for personal health.

IS HEALTH COACHING ACCESSIBLE? WHO WILL PAY FOR THIS?

The biggest challenge with supporting people to make foundational lifestyle health behavior changes is that there is no way to patent this model. The truth is that the foundations of health are simple. The health coaching model is more about the relationship between the coach and the patient and the communication tools that the coach uses to help the patient see how she might be in her own way, or might need to strengthen her boundaries or take some stressors off of her plate. This is not a quick fix, high profit medication, therapeutic technique, supplement, or surgery. It's a deep process of change. So, there is little motivation in our current model for making this transformation when no one can make billions of dollars a year from promoting it.

In 2019, the worldwide pharmaceutical market was worth nearly $1.3 trillion (Letter, 2020). That's a lot of profit to give up if clinicians and patients take back the healing system and prescribe and eat more broccoli and less sugar instead of metformin, which is prescribed nearly eighty million times each year in the US alone (Mikulic, 2020). At an average cost of $16.35, that represents over $1.3 billion in annual revenue.

You can see why the resistance to this change is strong. There are major stakeholders making a lot of money from keeping both clinicians and patients alike sick, tired, and struggling.

The health insurance industry also has a lot to lose in this transformation. Less need for healthcare means lower premiums as people realize they don't need as much medical intervention to stay healthy. One surprising outcome of the coronavirus pandemic is that while people stayed out of the healthcare system during the peak of the pandemic in New York, most did well despite getting less healthcare.

"As stay-at-home orders ease and cities reopen for business, many doctors and hospital administrators are calling for a quick return of health care to pre-pandemic levels. For months now, routine care has been postponed. Elective procedures – big money-makers – were halted so that hospitals could divert resources to treating COVID-19 patients. Routine clinic visits were canceled or replaced by online sessions. This has resulted in grievous financial losses for hospitals and clinics. Medical practices have closed. Hospitals have been forced to furlough employees or cut pay. Most patients, on the other hand, at least those with stable chronic conditions, seem to have done reasonably well. In a recent survey, only one in ten respondents said their health or a family member's health had worsened as a result of delayed care. Eighty-six percent said their health had stayed about the same, according to Dr. Sandeep Jauhar." (Jauhar, 2020).

The top health insurers profited over $35 billion in 2019. That's a lot to lose. Right now, while CPT billing codes are available for health coaching, it's not covered by most insurers. Thus, there is certainly inequality related to social determinants of health that limits access to health coaching to those who could benefit the most. As we transform the paradigm, this key factor must be kept at the forefront of the conversation.

Fortunately, the health coaching industry is continuing to press forward despite this resistance. Because we are at the beginning of this paradigm shift, those who don't adapt will be left behind. With little incentive for pharmaceutical companies or insurers to encourage this model, smaller tech companies and employers wanting to lower astronomical healthcare costs are pushing for change.

Consider Hinge Health. Hinge Health is a

company that sells physical therapy programs designed by physical therapists and delivered by health coaches directly to employers to lower their costs related to back and other joint pain. According to the Centers for Disease Control and Prevention (CDC), back pain costs employers $1,685 per employee every year. By focusing on foundational health skills including movement, sleep, and nutrition, Hinge Health can help employers lower those costs while keeping their employees healthier. Investors are seeing that this is the future of healthcare. Since 2014, Hinge Health, a small start-up with just over 200 employees, has raised over $150 million in funding.

What does this mean for your personal transformation from your clinical mindset to a coaching mindset? First, it means that there will be more job opportunities in the future for clinicians who take this leap in perspective and become highly trained, board-certified health coaches. Plus, it means that the opportunity is great for you to get creative if you're ready to create your own health coaching practice or side hustle. There has never been a better time for you to build the practice that allows you to help people achieve root cause healing and reach their health and life goals while optimizing your own health and energy. You can practice from anywhere (one of our Master Coaches lived on a boat for a year!). Your income potential is limitless (I now make more than seven times my original physical therapist annual salary). Your ability to design leveraged health models to serve low-income and other underserved populations is limitless (another of our Master Coaches runs a non-profit, public-private partnership program in a low-income population that helped its participants reduce their hemoglobin A1C by an average of a full point in just a few months!). And, best of all, your schedule is yours. This is your chance to work on your body's best schedule.

This is your chance to free yourself from the broken healthcare system and better serve your patients in the process.

References:

Jauhar S. People Have Stopped Going to the Doctor. Most Seem Just Fine. The New York Times. https://www.nytimes.com/2020/06/22/opinion/coronavirus-reopen-hospitals.html. Published June 22, 2020. Accessed September 26, 2020.
Letter TP. According to market research, the worldwide pharmaceutical market was worth nearly $1.3 trillion in 2019... TPL. https://www.thepharmaletter.com/article/annual-revenue-of-top-10-big-pharma-companies. Published March 3, 2020. Accessed September 26, 2020.
Mikulic M. Metformin hydrochloride prescriptions

number U.S. 2004-2017. Statista. https://www.statista.com/statistics/780332/metformin-hydrochloride-prescriptions-number-in-the-us/. Published January 2, 2020. Accessed September 26, 2020.

2

TAKE THE LEAP: TRANSFORM YOURSELF FROM CLINICIAN TO COACH

It was a beautiful summer day in 2011. I was walking around Brooklyn with my family, just hanging out, when my cell phone rang. It was one of my former patients from Houston. I had worked with her on her complex pelvic pain for several months as a physical therapist in a women's and pelvic health practice. We had gotten her pain stabilized, but it still flared almost every month at the time of her period. This had been going on for years. Finally, the patient was fed up and the doctors threw their hands up and recommended that she have a hysterectomy. She was about to have that surgery when she decided to try a recommendation I had given her a few months before, before I moved from Texas to the Northeast. I had, without much training or confidence, suggested that she try changing her diet to be less inflammatory. I suggested that she cut the dairy, gluten, sugar, and soy, eat more vegetables and see if that had any effect on her pain. It did.

As it turned out, living in Houston surrounded by Mexican restaurants, she would have queso cravings every month the few days before her period. Otherwise, she really didn't eat dairy, and her pain was well controlled. When she completely cut out the dairy, including her PMS cravings for cheese, her pain completely resolved. This simple change saved her from what would have been an ineffective hysterectomy which would have caused other problems with her health.

Working with that patient changed the trajectory of my practice.

She solidified the idea for me that simple interventions like dietary changes could have such a massive effect on complex conditions. She also taught me that the patient must take the leadership role in her care, that her day-to-day health behaviors can have a far greater effect than my ability to "fix" her pain.

That year, I embarked on the adventure of transforming my mindset and clinical practice completely from clinician to coach. To this day, I still work with clients clinically, making recommendations and helping them to collaborate with other health professionals to make decisions about their options around health behaviors and healing treatments, but now I start with the expectation that the client has the capacity to heal herself. I am there to hold the space for her to allow her to do so in community with people who support her in her life and on her health-care professional team.

WHERE IT ALL BEGIN

In 2011, I dove into building a health coaching practice in earnest. That year, I set up shop in a small, three-season porch in the back of my house. The small room contained little more than a card table, a tripod, a video camera, and a laptop. I eventually added a small heater when winter came.

At the time, I was driven by the mission to help women to see their own ability to heal themselves using the simple tools of small, day-by-day steps: changes in their nutrition, changes in their mindfulness practices, changes in their sleep behaviors, and changes in their exercise habits. What I learned was that, most of the time, women know the next step they need to take to improve their health, but they often lack the ability to take that step. Sometimes they really are too busy...working full time with four small children, a long commute, and a husband that travels for work. But, usually, there are internal barriers they must overcome before they can claim their health and make the health changes they need to make consistently, like feelings of unworthiness, poor emotional boundaries, or fears of risk or change. What I learned was that, by combining the clinical skills of functional nutrition, physical therapy, and lifestyle medicine with the communication skills that support women to overcome their barriers to change, my clients were experiencing more complete healing than I had ever before witnessed in my practice. This true integrative medicine was hard work for both of us, but it was magical.

Working with my first few clients in those early years when I was learning these skills, testing their efficacy, and integrating them in practice from 2009–2011 was a time of exploration for me. I had recently recovered from my own health challenges and was still in progress with my own implementation of consistent day-to-day health optimization behaviors. I had restored my health by this time and was finally able to have a second baby (seven years and a miscarriage later) of my own. I began my health coaching practice concurrent with the pregnancy, birth, and recovery of my second daughter. It was a time of deep transformation for me on all levels. And I was grateful that I had discovered a work opportunity that would stretch my mind while allowing me to work in an upstairs office, running down to nurse my baby whenever she needed me instead of trying to squeeze in a pumping session at my desk in the hospital.

When I started my practice, time flexibility was

extremely important to me. As a new mother of two girls, I still had a lot of ambition and care for my patients, but I also had new priorities to be more present with them in their lives. Small moments of presence throughout the day with my girls felt essential. Plus, I was much more aware of my need to take care of my own health after my burnout and health crash back in 2004, which lasted years before I began to find a path to healing. I was, and still am, committed to never going back to that level of sickness, anxiety, and fatigue if I have any say in the matter.

So, I spent a few years learning some new skills and becoming certified in health coaching while I was nursing. At the same time, I was deepening my own study of the evidence base for functional nutrition and lifestyle medicine interventions, such as sleep and the impacts of stress on health. I worked with several clients based on word-of-mouth conversations with my friends using mobile and telehealth models.

Then, in 2011, I went all in. I set up shop in that three-season porch with my laptop and a strong desire to help and took the leap from being in clinical practice to starting my own health coaching practice. It worked out perfectly! I had clients coming out of my ears right away, they all made weekly incredible transformations and found deeper states of healing than any of us thought possible. My professional peers were amazed by my practice results and couldn't wait to learn more about what I was doing!

Hahaha! Just kidding! It didn't happen like that at all.

Yes, the clients that I did work with made phenomenal progress. But it was a lot of work, blood, sweat, and tears on their part, and the humbling commitment to learning and practicing new coaching communication skills on my part. I worried about their progress; I was constantly unsure that these simple healthy lifestyle behaviors could really bring about such massive health improvements. And yet, often they did. I was also constantly criticized at that time, mostly by a few of my loudest peers in rehab, but sometimes by random doctors or college professors on Twitter. Some even threatened to "turn me in to my board." Many thought that I shouldn't be talking about things like nutrition and sleep. I was a physical therapist, and my critics often threatened to try to have my license revoked.

Plus, while I had those few word-of-mouth clients, I did not have a stable practice. I had no marketing plan or business plan, yet I was working harder than I ever had in the clinic. Plus, I made very little revenue and essentially no profit for years.

One of the best decisions I made that very first year that I decided to get serious about building this practice was that I hired a friend of mine who I knew from a mother-baby group that I was in with my oldest child. Her name is Nadja Lancaster. She was the organization to my mad scientist grand ideas. For years I paid her more than I paid myself, and it was well worth it! She is still with me today and is a key part of why my practice is so successful.

The other thing that I did right that first year that eventually paid off was to invest in marketing training, and business coaching. The sciences of business, sales, and marketing were foreign to me. I don't come from an entrepreneurial background, and this was my first venture into business. Even if you already have a business coach, join our program at The Integrative Women's Health Institute. This is the most valuable thing you can do wherever you are in your business journey. Most clinicians don't naturally love business. I sure didn't. But, if we're going to lead this transformation in healthcare, we must embrace the fact that healthcare is a business, and we must not shy away from learning and innovating this business if we're going to save ourselves and our clients from the destructive practices of most healthcare organizations today.

CHOOSING MY NICHE

2011 was the year that I got serious about building not only my own health coaching practice, but helping my colleagues make this shift as well. I knew from my own experience with intense sickness and recovery that this method of coaching combined with integrative practice was sorely needed in the world of women's health, complex chronic pain, and fatigue. That year, The Integrative Women's Health Institute was born. Actually, it was then called The Integrative Pelvic Health Institute, but I refined its focus a few years later with a mission to serve women.

From the start, I had a global vision, and I had a lot of hustle. I also knew that with hundreds of millions of women around the world with chronic pelvic pain alone – not to mention other hormone health issues, female athlete issues, and other common women's health concerns – I couldn't reach all of these women on my own. From the beginning, The Integrative Women's Health Institute was a place for women to come seeking their own healing and a place for practitioners to come for both education and their own healing. My coaching practice was always the research arm of my teaching institute. So, we tested everything to find the models that helped our clients to get their best results.

If you've ever heard me speak on the topic of practice building, I always emphasize the importance of choosing a narrow niche for your practice. This is key! But it took me a few tries to land on the kind of practice that I most enjoyed and that the world most needed.

I always had a clinical interest in women's and pelvic health, and specifically in chronic pelvic pain. This had been my focus for the twelve years of clinical practice up to that point, but what I really wanted to do was go upstream. I wanted to work with teenage girls right around the time of puberty or just a few years later, when most of the complex pelvic pain issues tend to begin. In fact, the number one reason that girls miss school in middle and high school is due to the pelvic pain related to endometriosis. It was important to me that instead of waiting until these women were in their thirties or forties, which is when I was seeing them in my word-of-mouth practice, that I tried to be very deliberate and go upstream and meet tween and teen girls as soon as they began dealing with period issues. I knew that my gynecologist colleagues didn't have a lot of tools for them at the time. All they were trained to do was to recommend hormonal birth control or pain medications as band aids for the symptoms.

So, I dove in with big ideas for reaching teens before they had to suffer from prolonged problems of pain, infertility, and hormonal imbalances later in life! I developed marketing materials and a signature talk that I presented all around the New York City area near where I was living at the time. I began to focus my marketing efforts on working with teen girls and their parents. It was great! There was definitely a need for this. Once word got around that this was what I was doing, parents were flocking to me for help. I once hosted a live workshop at my local library on the topic of tweens, teens, and periods, told about six people about it, and sixty moms showed up! I met a dad on the train that brought his wife and daughter to my office the next week for help. *But…*it turned out I was not yet experienced with working with teenage girls, and I underestimated what it would take to engage them and their families. Don't get me wrong, I adore teen girls. I just didn't have the skills to support them yet. Working with teens requires a special ability to work with the girls and their whole families. That same dad who rushed in to see me with his wife and daughter was unwilling to eat more vegetables himself in support and solidarity with his daughter. It takes a special person to work in pediatrics, and I was not one of those people. I should have known this, since I never once worked with peds in my entire clinical career to that point, never even did a three-month rotation in peds. Thus, I refocused my practice on adult women with pelvic pain. And, in the meantime also developed my skills to work better with teens so that later I could successfully expand into working with teen girls. My personal experience years later of being a mom of tween and teen girls also deeply informed my practice.

But that experience taught me an essential business lesson. If you want to be a leader in the transformation of the healthcare system, you must put yourself out there and try things in real life with people, not alone in your office in your own head. Everything in business is a test, and you won't know how well you did until you try it with other people out in the world. Choosing your niche is essential, but you can't do it in a vacuum.

BUILDING THE HEALING TRANSFORMATION CONTAINER

In addition to clarifying your niche - who you want to help and what problem you want to help them solve, you'll also need to figure out how to build the best container to support your ideal client to reach their goals. This is a foreign concept for most health professionals, because up until now, you've likely worked in or built the kind of practice that is familiar to you. Someone calls a front desk, makes an appointment, sees you for that visit, hopes to make some progress, and maybe comes back and sees you again to follow up sometime in the future. This goes on as long as it takes until your patient is ready to be discharged out into the world, or they just stop coming.

In the new healthcare model, your opportunities to create a wide variety of healing, transformative containers is vast. You get to consider how you like to work, where you like to work, how much time it tends to take for people in your niche to see progress, how they are best supported, and more! When you start reinventing the models for healing, you can come up with some pretty creative things.

After testing our endometriosis coaching program for about seven years, we have come up with the following model:

- Our clients do best when starting with a four-month commitment to their own health.
- Before they even start the program, they meet with me for a thirty-minute strategy session to see if they are ready for help, they want to invest the time and energy to work on their health now, and if we want to do it together.
- Then, the client meets with my team for a one-hour introductory session to help her to map out her personalized plan with a functional nutrition practitioner, leading with the coaching perspective that she already knows a lot about what strategies do and don't work for her while staying

open to ideas that she may not have
considered before.

- Over the following four months, she will
  meet approximately weekly with a health
  coach on our team to keep overcoming the
  barriers in her life and her mind that are
  keeping her from making big changes in
  her health behaviors day-in and day-out.

- And, during that time, she will also meet
  with her functional nutrition professional
  and other members of her professional
  healing team to get input, ideas, and
  professional consultation about the
  healing strategies that she's implementing
  with her coach.

- We also track data across those four months,
  including tracking scores on validated
  outcome measures, gut microbiome
  composition, blood sugar stability, heart rate
  variability, and graphic perspectives on how
  her physical systems are healing over time
  from a functional nutrition perspective.

After their initial four-month commitment, some
clients stay with us for years for support and clinical
conversations with a focus on new goals like being
able to reach more physical challenges like running a
local race, hiking across Europe, getting pregnant, or

recovering postpartum. The goals can always expand. There is always more to work towards as long as the client would like to keep expanding. Sometimes maintenance support for a while, when things feel good to her, is also a great idea.

But that's just our endometriosis coaching program container. Our Integrative Women's Health Institute graduates have built beautiful containers of their own meeting their unique needs and the needs of their unique niche clients. Casie Danenhauer built her own private practice that includes local and destination retreats, including with another of our brilliant grads, Brianne Grogan. Brianne partnered with Casie for their global pelvic health retreat, and she maintains a massive digital presence supporting women in every corner of the world with her FemFusion Fitness YouTube channel. Vashti Kanahele, living in the middle east, partnered with Lisa Arendell, living in Louisiana, to bring a digital and telehealth coaching container to women around the world who are recovering from breast explant surgery. Caroline Zwickson created the signature Well Mama program using a digital platform. She supports new mothers in reclaiming their physical and mental health while deepening their connection with their partners to improve their parenting. This is life changing work that can affect the health of families across generations.

Dr. Naja Chikazunga-Martin leads with health

coaching and nutrition in her pelvic physical therapy practice. When her schedule is too busy to fit in a new client, she supports them digitally with lifestyle changes for them to implement in the interim before they can see her in person or via telehealth. Dr. Chikazunga-Martin is changing lives every day with this innovative container, improving her clinical outcomes and reducing her burnout. As her client, thirty-seven-year-old Termeca Mitchell, said, "I'm a mother of three who has been struggling with pelvic pain for years. After having numerous surgeries, I finally thought I was fixed. But in 2017, I began having pelvic pain again, so I scheduled an appointment to see my doctor. He stated that I was fine, so I went about my day. As time passed, the pain started to get worse, so I scheduled another appointment with my doctor, but he wasn't in. I was told I had to see another doctor, who told me that it was normal to have pains in my pelvic area because, even though I had a partial hysterectomy, my body still had the symptoms of a menstrual cycle and that I still ovulate. After that appointment, I thought, 'Maybe that's true,' and just brushed it off. Long story short, the pain began to be unbearable to the point where it interfered with work and my daily activities.

"My husband and I decided to schedule an appointment with my doctor who performed the surgery. After seeing him, I was scheduled to do pelvic therapy with Naja. When I met with her, she talked with me and sent me an email with a nourishment guide I should try. Due to scheduling conflicts, I missed a couple of appointments but thought, *Hey, let me try this diet thing*. So I started on the diet Naja sent. During the first week or so into the process, I started to feel so much better, and in six weeks, my pain had decreased. I am now able to perform house chores and have intercourse without pain. I saw Naja for my second visit and was excited to share with her that I had begun an exercise routine of two to three times per week and was enjoying intercourse with no pain." This client's life was literally changed, her marriage improved, and she even got a new job all because Naja shifted her perspective and remained open to her own innovative ideas, allowing her to create the perfect container for healing for her unique client population. Each of our graduates uniquely represents what's possible in re-imaging healthcare by thinking outside the box of the traditional healthcare practice model.

In the next chapter, join me as we walk through the process of how you can build your own transformative coaching practice.

3

EXPAND YOUR OPPORTUNITIES: THE CLINICIAN TO COACH METHOD

The process of transforming your practice from clinician to coach is simple, but it requires commitment to each step in the process, skill development, practice, mentorship, and coaching to support you to keep progressing, and a willingness to step outside of your comfort zone. In the following chapters, I will share the process with you in detail. For now, let's review the steps and their optimal order of progression.

As you start your transformation from clinician to coach, step one will be to make a significant shift in how you communicate with your patients. You can begin this stage even before you've made the leap to starting a coaching practice by practicing this skill with your current patients or clients, and even friends and family members. The communication perspective that you were likely taught in your clinical education was an educator or expert perspective. Your role was to listen to your patient, listen for clues to her diagnosis or functional impairments, and then, based on your training combined with the pattern recognition gained from your clinical experience, give her therapeutic recommendations. With this perspective, you didn't really get her to buy into the process or ask her what she thinks her next step in her healing process should be. You didn't ask her why she may or may not be able to implement your recommendations in her daily life or about any anticipated barriers to her making the changes you recommended. Essentially, you assessed her situation using your clinical training and experience and told her what to do to heal. Sometimes this works well, but it's a clinical perspective on communication, it's not coaching. Thus, step one in the clinician to coach method is to learn, understand, and practice coaching communication skills. In essence, these skills are opposite from how you communicate now and will feel like a foreign language at first. You'll learn to think in questions instead of recommendations, and you'll learn to speak and listen in a way that engages your patient differently. You'll also learn the power of anticipating barriers to change, and how to use your client's past successes and failures in other areas of her life to apply to helping her make these health behavior changes. You'll learn the details of this transition in the next chapter.

In Chapter 5, you'll begin to lay the foundation for your successful practice. Your practice will not be financially successful if you don't master the skills in that chapter. Chapter 5 will teach you how to identify and refine your ideal client. Your entire marketing strategy and business development strategy, in terms of which integrative health and coaching skills you need to develop and what experience to gain with patients and clients, hinges on this step in the process. Not only will your practice fail financially, but you won't be able to help your clients get the best outcomes possible if you don't commit to this step. If you're like most of our health coach certification students, you will resist this step. You'll be challenged to narrow your ideal client enough. You'll worry about leaving people out that you can help. No need to worry about either of these issues. Suspend disbelief, and consider Chapter 5 with a beginner's mind.

In Chapter 6, you'll learn the importance of building community as an essential part of your marketing strategy and potentially your coaching practice. In Chapter 5, you'll have detailed your niche and ideal client. Some niche markets thrive on a community aspect to their healing process. For example, postpartum women meeting in a group coaching format not only progress along their own healing paths, but are often going through similar things. The opportunity for peer support, encouragement, and motivation are strong in groups like this who are making significant life transformations as a part of their healing. While some niches are not as conducive to healing in group coaching containers, they will still benefit from a community aspect in your content marketing. When there is a lot of engagement during your live videos, community events, or even on your Instagram page, your potential clients – who are going through similar challenges – feel a sense of "not being alone" that is powerful to their healing whether or not they enroll in your paid programs.

Chapters 7 and 8 are all about the foundational skills of functional nutrition and lifestyle medicine. If your goal is to build a health coaching practice, distinct from a life or business coaching practice, you must commit to developing your expertise in foundational health skills. What you probably didn't learn in your clinical education program was that health is skillset, not a destination. Most clinical education programs emphasize the most complex health interventions without optimizing foundational health skills such as good sleep, nutrient dense anti-inflammatory nutrition, recovery, support and stress balance, and movement. These foundational skills seem exceedingly simple. Don't your clients already know these things? Maybe, but most are not implementing them regularly. Plus, there is some degree of complexity to it once the foundation is set. Sometimes the simple health skills are not enough to unravel years of experiencing a chronic condition, and you'll need to educate your client on options such as functional laboratory testing, supplementation, therapeutic diets, advanced sleep optimization strategies, or personalized exercise interventions. This piece of the puzzle is fascinating to most clinicians, but remember, these steps must not supersede the previous steps in The Clinician to Coach Method, otherwise you'll risk slipping back into the clinical mindset and method of communication.

Finally, in Chapter 9, you'll learn the details of creating the best coaching container and method for both you and your ideal client. This is the key to transforming the burnout culture of modern healthcare. It's likely you don't have to see fifteen or more patients in a day and put most of your attention on productivity billing for the sake of the organization's profitability. Your clients don't need to be rushed through telling their health stories, being interrupted within the first eleven seconds of sharing their insights on their own health. Creating the right coaching container and process for both you and your clients will allow you to serve your clients well to reach their health goals in the easiest and most supportive possible way for all of you. Deep consideration, mentoring, and taking action on this step will allow you to bring your coaching practice vision into reality. Transforming your practice process will empower your patients to own their healing, completing your transformation from clinical "mechanic" to encouraging guide.

Now that you understand the process of transformation from clinician to coach, let's get started!

4

HEALTH COACHING SKILLS FOR HEALTH TRANSFORMATION

Committing to mastery of the skills of health coaching communication is key to your transformation and the transformation of your practice from the top down, recommendation-focused, high-stress clinical model to using an integrative approach led with a coaching mindset.

WHAT IS HEALTH COACHING?

How is health coaching different from clinical health care? The key to transitioning from a clinical mindset to a coaching mindset is that you will begin to both think differently and communicate differently with your patients, clients, and colleagues.

The National Board of Health and Wellness Coaches is the international health coach training approval organization that oversees the health coach board exam internationally. According to their definition, "Health and wellness coaches partner with clients seeking *self-directed* lasting changes, aligned with their values, which promote health and wellness and thereby enhance wellbeing. In the course of their work, health and wellness coaches display unconditional positive regard for their clients and a belief in their capacity for change and honoring that each client is an expert on his or her life while ensuring that all interactions are respectful and non-judgmental." Health coaching is the process that creates a bridge between knowing what to do for your health and actually doing it. According to The International Coach Federation, 98 percent of coaching clients report that working with a coach was a positive decision and worth the expense. People are very happy to coach and be coached because it's always such a positive self-growth experience, even when it is challenging and difficult.

The key to transforming your practice to lead with a coaching mindset is to master the skills of health coach communication. Combine this powerful method of communication with integrative, evidence-based healing recommendations, and you will have a powerfully effective, successful practice.

Health coaching includes the coaching communication skills that are very similar to business coaching or life coaching or any other kind of coaching, but the educational component, the informational component, is about lifestyle medicine. It's about optimizing someone's root core foundations of health – their nutrition, their sleep, their movement and exercise, mindfulness, stress management, support networks, and so forth. Health coaching holds the expectation that the client has innate wisdom to understand her best next step for healing, though she may need support, education, and resources to understand her options.

Health coaches have the communication skills to inspire consistent, long term health behavior change. And they collaborate with and are a part of the healing team that helps each client figure out which individual behavior changes are most important for them to make in which priority order. It is primarily the role of the coach to help each client elicit her internal health wisdom. We, as human beings, have some idea and understanding, based on our own experiences and knowledge, what we need to do to stay healthy. We know we need to sleep, and usually we know when we are tired; we have some educated guesses about what kinds of foods we should eat and exercise we should do. While our clients may often need more education or more clinical intervention to figure out exactly what nutrition, exercise, or sleep program to follow, most of our clients have good guesses about their best next steps for healing.

Health coaching is a fierce commitment to your client's health and life goals. You don't let her give up on herself. As coaches, we take a stand for our clients, which includes a little bit of tough love and a lot of bravery. We are challenged to hold our clients accountable when they give up on themselves, when they change their minds or try to quit. When your client says, "Oh, this is getting too hard" is exactly when she needs you the most.

HOLDING SPACE

The best health coaches bravely hold space to allow their clients to sit with and feel their emotions. Think about holding space as creating an environment of pure space, a container where someone can tell their story, share their fears, and freely express their challenges. This is their safe space to talk about the things they need to overcome to reach their health goals and do the vulnerable work to figure out how to overcome their barriers to change. Their emotions and fears can be vulnerably placed into the space knowing that the coach in the space with them is not going to judge them for it. She is going to help them work through it and sit with their emotions about making this healing change without judgement. It's literally a place of calm to safely express anything your client needs to share. Your job is to create a beautiful container with your energy, where your client feels safe and supported.

TRUSTING THAT YOUR CLIENT KNOWS HER BEST NEXT STEP

How is health coaching different from clinical health-care? In health coaching we trust that the client usually already knows the next right step to take. Most people know, for example, that they should be eating vegetables, not Oreos, and yet…thus, usually our clients know their best next step towards optimal health (sometimes they really don't, and get confused or stuck. We'll get to that later).

Usually, even when your client knows that her pain will improve if she eats less processed food and more vegetables, goes to bed earlier, walks outdoors each day, and so on, often she's simply not doing those things. Thus, though your client likely knows at least the next best step in her journey to optimal, she's probably not taking that step consistently. With a coaching mindset, even if education or thera-peutic recommendations are needed, each action step is ultimately chosen by the client, sometimes with intervention, education, and/or resources from the coach. Healing requires taking action. It is not a passive event.

Most people know that, to improve their energy, they should stop eating sugar and eat more vegeta-bles. That's not earth shattering. Supporting your clients to actually take that action is your main work when you begin to take on a coaching mindset to health. We transform from putting most of our energy into making skilled clinical recommendations to helping our clients to actually take consistent action and an active role, whether they are healing from an injury or illness or optimizing their day-to-day health.

WHEN YOUR CLIENT IS CONFUSED

Now, there is certainly a role for clinically skilled intervention, and evidence-based health education in your work with clients. Sometimes our clients really don't know what the best next step is for her to take. Should she be on a vegan diet or keto? Should she intermittent fast or eat every few hours? Should she run or lift weights? Sometimes our clients really are confused. So, don't throw the baby out with the bathwater. While we'll be leading with a coaching mindset, there is a place for your skilled health education and recommendations. But start with coaching. Don't rush through this. Take time in the space you hold with your clients, and use the tools of health coaching to be very sure that she needs your skilled input before giving it to her. It's essential that you trust the coaching process, and that prioritizes trusting your client's intuition, strengthening her ability to trust herself.

Eventually, you may support her in her exploration of clinical options to help her determine her next healing step. You can offer clinical recommendations in collaboration with her based on your expertise. You can help her to explore her options, research, and see other practitioners. Then, the decision is in her hands, her mind, and her intuition, which you help her to navigate in that safe space. Be present, support her in thinking about all of the clinical options including the risks and benefits, and then ask, "What does your intuition say?" Then, the client will make her next step decision, which is always open to modification. Then, your role is to fiercely hold her accountable to herself. This is your role when she starts to stumble, and thinks, "Oh, this is getting too hard, I don't want to do this anymore." You'll reply, "Do you really not want to do this anymore, or is it just getting too hard?" This is the real work.

Lead with the expectation that your client already knows the best next step. Trust that there's a lot that she already knows. Your trust in her helps her to build her trust in herself. Hold space for her to deepen her trust in her own innate healing wisdom, and be a resource for skilled exploration of her clinical options.

We'll talk more about how to consider her clinical options by combining your clinical expertise with an integrative approach and evidence-based lifestyle medicine in Chapters 7 and 8.

IS YOUR CLIENT READY TO TRANSFORM?

Is your client ready to make the changes required to optimize her health? Initially anyone making any change will be in the pre-contemplation stage. This is where someone has no intention of changing their behavior. "Yes, I'm a smoker. I don't think it's affecting my health at all. I don't care. I'm not going to stop smoking. I don't care what you say." That's representative of the pre-contemplation stage.

The next step is contemplation. "All right, I'm aware that smoking is not good for me. People have been telling me that forever. I understand that intellectually, but I'm not interested in quitting smoking now."

Preparation is the next stage. "Okay, I understand that smoking is not good for my health. I'm ready to start thinking about addressing this problem, but first I need to think about what all of my different options are for smoking cessation programs."

Taking action is the next stage. In this stage, someone has chosen *how* they're going to change their behavior. "I've chosen a particular smoking cessation program, and I'm ready to start it."

Maintenance is the next stage. This is the time to solidify and sustain the change. At this point, your client will be thinking, "Now I am a person who doesn't smoke. I've made a transformation from a person who smokes to a person who doesn't smoke."

Your client might still need some support at this time to maintain that change during trigger times when someone might slip into old behavior patterns, such as smoking when out with friends who smoke or during stressful times.

Ideally, for your coaching engagement to be the most successful, your client will at least be in the contemplation phase. But there are some advanced strategies to help people progress from pre-contemplation through to action.

THE COACHING PROCESS

The process of coaching starts with a commitment to the process for both client and coach. You'll start with a program agreement, which we'll discuss further in Chapter 9. This formal commitment to the process over the course of a defined period of time is essential for helping your client to overcome her barriers to change when things get difficult. The program agreement underlies and defines the professional coaching relationship. Then, the client will kick off the program by defining her vision of success, so that both client and coach know the client's vision and goals for the process and remain committed to that vision, even when taking action to change her health behaviors gets challenging.

THE COACHING RELATIONSHIP

The professional coaching relationship requires a commitment to the client's vision, whether or not the coach would have the same goals if she were in the client's position. It also requires that the focus of every session remains on the client. Commonly, coaches can empathize with what their client is going through and will have a desire to share a story from her own life. Usually, that's not helpful. The goal is to keep the focus nearly entirely on the client, and her unique story, actions, mindset, and challenges. Plus, when the process is client-led and the attention is maintained on the client overcoming her unique obstacles, then the pressure to "fix" is removed from the client/coach relationship. Changing those dynamics, from the clinician-coach being responsible for "fixing" the client to the client being responsible for naming her goals, working with the coach on each next step health behavior, working with the coach to overcome her obstacles to behavior change, making space for action, taking action, and celebrating her successes shifts the dynamic of responsibility from the clinician (coach) to the client. This is extremely liberating for the clinician-coach and the client alike. Our students constantly share with us how just changing this dynamic vastly reduces their feelings of burnout immediately. Plus, the client gets better results faster and is more empowered in the process.

The coaching relationship is a professional relationship with defined terms based on the program agreement. This is not a friendship. You are strongly advised not to coach your family members or close friends. A coaching relationship is distinct, and you may hold back from getting your client a depth of possible results if you don't have that professional distance. Close friends or family members should be referred to your colleagues. Fortunately, in our community at The Integrative Women's Health Institute, you'll have the opportunity to meet thousands of wonderful, skilled coaches who practice in a wide variety of niches all over the world.

Coaching is not primarily health education, consultation, or skilled therapeutic recommendations. While all of those skills do play a role in health coaching, I am going to challenge you right here not to lean on your comfort zone in these areas. Instead, challenge yourself to develop your coaching skills before bringing in your more established skills of health education, consultation, and therapeutic recommendations and interventions. This will feel difficult at first because it's almost the opposite of what you learned in your clinical training, but this is the key to minimizing your burnout while getting more lasting, root cause resolving healing for your clients. Don't give up!

Health coaching does overlap with psychotherapy, but it is not the same thing. Psychotherapists focus on mental health conditions listed in the DSM-5. They focus on assessment, diagnosis, and treatment of mental disorders. Both health coaches and psychotherapists work with clients with issues related to chronic illness, post-op states, general wellness, self-care issues, and stress. Both use interpersonal relationships as a healing modality, both use behavior change strategies and may have similar goals.

Health coaching utilizes tools and skills from psychology research. Health coaching is an evidence-based practice based on tools and skills for behavior change, transformation and sustained action. The various theoretical frameworks and conceptual models used in coaching such as self-determination theory, adult development theory, learning theory, motivational interviewing, social cognitive theory, and so forth are concepts and theories that are used in health coaching that are based on psychology literature. Both psychology and coaching use research from the fields of cognitive behavioral therapy, positive psychology, and neuroscience.

Psychologists work with clients who struggle with mental instability. The psychotherapist's patient's level of instability, anxiety, or tension is so high as to be destructive to the person's ability to function. Therapy seeks to comfort the afflicted so that they can continue to progress and excel in society and meet their life's goals. There's a focus on safety. Keeping the person safe so that she can function. Coaches work with mentally stable clients in an environment of safety and trust, but coaches are called upon to afflict the comfortable. We seek to help our clients to move out of stable and safe-feeling mindsets and behaviors to be open to new insights, understandings, and actions. Creating the space such that your client feels it's okay, or even good, to feel uncomfortable is key to helping them move from a limiting comfort zone to a new comfort zone (that at first feels uncomfortable), so that they can make the changes required to meet their goals. We're stretching people who are comfortable, but need to be stretched in order to become happier and healthier.

For example, imagine you're working with a client who, as a part of her vision, would like to reduce or relieve her chronic pain so that she can hike in Yosemite National Park with her family this summer. One of her action steps is to eliminate gluten, dairy, sugar, and soy from her diet as a goal towards relieving her pain. At first, making this daily change in her diet might feel hard. She has to learn uncomfortable new ways to cook, order differently at restaurants, overcome her fear of being seen as high maintenance, and learn new strategies for coping with sadness instead of eating ice cream to dull her emotional pain. All of these shifts will be uncomfortable. But with your coaching support, she'll move from her comfort zone of eating her prior less healthy (but low maintenance and emotionally soothing) diet to her new comfort zone of eating her healthier (pain-relieving) diet, celebrating the fact that she had to overcome many challenges for this to become a new habit.

That said, there are some clients who are not appropriate for coaching, and many red flags to be aware of for referral and/or collaboration with other health professionals on the team. We cover this in a lot of depth in our health coaching certification program, but here are a few examples: hostile behavior or the client bullying you. If your client displays unrelenting anger, excessive anger or resentment, reckless or impulsive behavior, and so on these are behavioral red flags. There are physical red flags too, such as complaints of acute lack of sleep, somatic disorders, or symptoms of unresolved or prolonged grief. Not all clients with these red flags are not appropriate for coaching, but if they display these red flags, they may need clinical intervention from you or another healthcare professional on her team before she is ready for coaching or collaboratively with the coaching engagement.

As a health professional, establishing the professionalism of this relationship from the start is essential to your client's success and ultimately, to her autonomy. As Abraham Lincoln once said, "Commitment is what transforms a promise into a reality. It's the stuff character is made of. It's the power to change the face of things. It's the daily triumph of integrity over skepticism." From Day One of the coaching relationship, be clear about your role as the coach, and be sure that she understands her role as the client. She will be the one setting the vision and goals, clearing space in her life to take action, taking the action, and owning and celebrating the achievements along her healing journey.

VISION

Why does she want to be so healthy? What if there were no limits to what's possible for her? What does that look like? What does success look like to her? What emotions come up when considering a limitless vision? What does her ideal health or life look like by her definition? There are so many different versions of what someone wants their health to look like and what she wants to be healthy for, it's not for us, as coaches, to define. Your client's vision, by her definition, is the vision you will take a stand for, even if it's not something you would ever come up with.

Maybe she wants to backpack around the world hitting all of the major bungee jumping spots. You would never in a million years want to do that, or even advise it. That's fine. This is not your vision. It's essential that you stay focused on her desires, whether or not you agree with them (if you disagree strongly, she is not the right client for you as you won't be able to fiercely take a stand for her vision).

MINDFULNESS AND MINDFUL LISTENING

Mindfulness is simply awareness of the present moment. Being aware of the present moment without judgment. Your mind will wander when you're holding space for people, your mind will judge what your clients say. Staying mindful when your mind wants to judge or be distracted will require you to practice mindfulness on a daily basis.

The benefits of a daily mindfulness practice for healers are vast. You will improve your ability to focus, be productive without burnout, be more creative, and have more energy for your work and everything else in your life. Not only will your mindfulness practice benefit you, it will also benefit your clients.

Give your clients a deep gift of safe, non-judgmental creative space for reflection, idea generation, and validation. Think about this for yourself; it's so rare to have this experience of being mindfully listened to. How would it feel to simply share your story with someone who will sit with you without rushing, without judgement, without advice for how to "fix" your pain? How would it feel to have the supported space to brainstorm your own ideas for your next healing step? To be fully supported to express your deepest goals and desires?

This is mindful listening.

Feeling listened to without judgement is healing in and of itself. Developing this skill to give to your clients takes commitment and daily practice to self-manage your own mind.

As clinicians, we are taught pattern recognition, and our brains start to do that pretty quickly when patients start telling us their stories. Instead, come to each client session with a beginner's mind, a complete openness to curiosity. Don't be attached to anything she's going to say and just be mindful of your own distractions, of your own thoughts wandering, of your own judgements, of your own pattern recognition, and notice how much work it is to literally do nothing but attentively listen. Notice how much self-managing you have to do of your own thoughts to be able to give your client this gift. As you develop this essential skill, you will become a far more effective healer. By enhancing your ability to transfer the work of healing to your client, you will enhance her autonomy and ability to deeply heal.

REFLECTIONS

When you give your client the space to share her own story of her health challenge, one skill to enhance your mindful listening is to reflect her story back to her. Because it's so challenging to get healthcare professionals and others to listen, our client will often have told their story over and over again in a loop to others and themselves. Sometimes clients get so numb to their own story that they barely realize what they are saying, and some of the story's essential truth gets lost.

Thus, "reflections" of your client's storytelling is a tool where you speak back to your client nearly exactly, in her words, a key point in the story that she just spoke to you. This technique does two things. First, the client gets a chance to step out of the loop in her head and decide whether or not what she just told you is true from her perspective, and it stops her looped thinking ,giving her the ability to powerfully own her story. She can then confirm that you really listened to and heard her, building trust in the relationship.

POWERFUL QUESTIONS

One of the biggest struggles that clinicians have when transforming from the clinician (recommendations/"fixing") mindset to the coaching (witnessing/holding accountable/supporting) mindset is to stop making recommendations and start thinking in questions. As your client is moving through the coaching process, she will often get stuck regarding what to do next. Your role as her coach is not to suggest what she should do next, but to keep asking her powerful questions to help her determine what to do next and then commit to taking that action.

Examples of powerful questions include:

- What do you think is your next right step in this process?
- What support do you need to take action?
- What will you do that is entirely in your power and not dependent on the actions or permissions of others?
- How will you create time in your day to add this exercise commitment to your schedule?
- How will you soothe your emotions when this (unhealthy behavior) is no longer an option?

INTERNAL/EXTERNAL BARRIERS TO CHANGE

Your client's barriers to change are the obstacles that have kept her from reaching her health and life goals without your support. These barriers can be external or practical, such as not knowing how to cook, having an inflexible work schedule, or having limited financial resources. The obstacles can be internal, such as fears around making the changes, embarrassment around making the changes, not wanting to make others feel bad, or having difficulty with maintaining healthy emotional boundaries. Helping your clients to bring awareness to their individual barriers to change is one of the most important parts of your work as a coach. Many people are simply blind to their own barriers to change until they commit to the coaching process and take the time to discover their own barriers.

OVERCOMING BARRIERS TO CHANGE

It's one thing to be aware of your boundaries, it's another thing for your clients to be ready and willing to overcome their barriers to change and then actually to break through those barriers. Overcoming barriers to change is the deep work of coaching. Once your client recognizes, for example, that she's giving her power away to her boss, friend, partner, or someone else, it can be difficult and scary to take it back. Building her physical and emotional strength, building webs of supportive people to help her, creating space in her schedule, and taking the action needed to take her power back is a process that takes time and consistent commitment. Ultimately, her health depends on her ability to recognize her barriers to making consistent health changes and then getting the support she needs to make those changes every day. Just as an example, imagine the impact in just one year of your client going from drinking very little water and two cups of coffee and one alcoholic drink every day to drinking no alcohol or caffeine and drinking nine cups of water daily. Even this one simple change would have a ripple effect reducing many common daily symptoms, including fatigue, pain, and more even after just a few weeks of consistent action. Why doesn't everyone make these simple daily changes? We all have barriers to change that we're not even aware of. Recognizing and then getting support and taking steps to overcome these barriers leads to amazing transformation, and the results can be surprisingly fast and simple. But the right support and accountability systems must be in place for these changes to be sustained and transformative.

CELEBRATION

Don't skip the celebration! Many of our clients have a "never enough" mentality. As soon as they overcome a barrier or achieve a goal, they are already thinking about what they need to do next. But, stopping to celebrate and learn lessons from each goal achievement will optimize your client's coaching experience. Sometimes taking lessons learned from success will power the next success even more quickly and easily.

MAINTENANCE AND GROWTH

The coaching process is lifelong. Optimal health is not a finish line, it's a lifelong process. As your clients achieve one health goal, often they have more goals on the horizon. There is always more living to do. Don't skip the celebrations along the way, but do keep supporting your clients to move to their next level of transformation. The game of life is filled with opportunities. Sometimes there are setbacks. The longer you immerse yourself in the work of coaching, the more you'll realize that life is an amazing journey, and having the health to reach for your unique goals makes it easier to weather the hard times and deeply enjoy the good times.

"IS MY FOCUS TOO NARROW?" THE SURPRISING BENEFITS OF FOCUSING ON ONE IDEAL CLIENT

Now that you have a better understanding of what the coaching process and the coaching mindset are, we're going to shift gears a bit and talk about setting the foundation of your coaching business. Of course, you will need to deepen and practice your coaching skills with mentorship and experience, and along the way, you want to be just as committed to learning the business and marketing skills that you will need to actually connect with clients who need your coaching. It doesn't do anyone any good if you're a brilliant coach and brilliant clinician who employs the most effective integrative healing tools if you don't have any clients to serve. In this chapter, I'm going to begin to teach you the foundational business and marketing skills you'll need.

One of the biggest struggles that new coaches

have is, "Where should I focus my marketing time, energy, and money when I'm just getting my practice started?" The first thing you have to figure out is who your service is for. Everything you create, your coaching program, your marketing messaging, your workshops, your social media posts, your entire marketing strategy must speak directly to the clients you want to serve. This is known as creating a niche practice. There are other ways to grow a coaching practice such as through networking and personal referrals, but the fastest and easiest way to grow a coaching practice is to create a niche practice.

What is a niche? Your niche is the type of clients that you serve to help them get the result that they want. For example, you might create a practice focused on helping new mothers resolve their challenges with postpartum incontinence. Or, you might build a practice focused on helping college track athletes recover from injuries more quickly and easily. You clarify your niche by clearly stating who you help and the result that you help them to achieve. That is your niche.

To take this a step further, you should know as much as possible about your ideal client. Literally think of her as one person. For your marketing strategy and your practice to be the most successful, you'll need to deeply understand your ideal client. You should be able to describe her in detail, and get to know her as well as a detailed character in a novel.

Ideally, she will be based on one person (or a combination of factors from a few people) that you would love to work with over and over again in your practice. Think of your favorite past client(s), and let's clone her into a character. You should know her as well as the author of a novel knows the main character in her story. You should be able to make predictions about her life. What movies she might enjoy, how she likes to consume information, things that would annoy her, who she would be friends with, etc.

Sample details to consider about your ideal client:

- Name
- Where she lives (city, suburban, or rural area)?
- Age and other relevant demographics
- Income level
- Occupation
- Schedule
- Things she would find funny
- Things that would annoy her
- Relationship status
- Children or pets
- Volunteer causes
- Hobbies
- Social butterfly or loner

Take some time to really get to know your ideal

client. Think of the details of her life. This will make everything you write to her in your marketing messaging so much easier.

Then, define the number one problem that you can help her to solve. This should be a problem that is so bothersome to her that she's googling it in the middle of the night. She's obsessed with solving it. Then, consider what the solution would look like to her. For example, your ideal client is a thirty-four-year-old working mother of a three-year-old. She works full time as a nurse in the NICU at a hospital and is struggling with intense anxiety and insomnia. It's now affecting her work, her sleep, and her sanity. She has tried everything she can think of to overcome it. She exercises nearly every day as a part of her training for the local triathlons she does on the weekends, she has tried sleeping medication, but she just can't seem to calm herself down and stay asleep all night. Her number one problem that she wants you to help her solve is her anxiety-related insomnia, and she is willing to do pretty much anything to solve it. The solution looks like being able to sleep calmly all night and feel relaxed, rested, and focused when she's at work and home in the evenings and weekends with her husband and daughter. She hates having to ask for help with this, but she has run out of ideas. She wants to solve this with you privately because she hates to admit she's even having this struggle.

Now that you know your ideal client so clearly, your marketing strategy is much easier. First, consider where your thirty-four-year-old working mom nurse triathlete ideal client with anxiety and insomnia might hang out? What she might listen to? Read? Watch?

- Working moms groups in person or online
- Moms of toddler or preschooler groups
- Nurse groups, communities, or conferences
- Facebook support groups for anxiety
- The Instagram pages of psychologists who specialize in anxiety
- Podcasts about sleep
- Blogs about parenting
- Nursing conferences or newsletters
- Weekend warrior triathlon clubs

Then, start writing articles, posts, filming videos, or creating other content to talk to your ideal client in the places where she hangs out. Map out a strategy that every quarter you will focus on one medium. For example, this quarter you will pitch ten podcast hosts each week to be interviewed on podcasts that your ideal client is most likely to listen to, such as podcasts on sleep, nursing, anxiety, triathlon training, or motherhood. The secret to successful marketing messaging that your ideal client will actually see is to write (or create audio or video) content that will interest her specifically and share it in places where she is likely to already be hanging out either in person or virtually.

When you are very clear on your ideal client and the problem that you can help her solve, it will be easy for you to attract clients to your practice. And, as a bonus, not only will your practice grow more easily from a business development standpoint, but you'll also become more and more skilled in your niche area. Having a specific specialty also allows you to focus your continued professional development on stronger coaching skills and integrative healing skills that will be the most useful for this specific client. If your practice is filled with women in their thirties who are struggling with anxiety and insomnia, there is no need to spend your valuable time deepening your skills in cancer recovery or any other of the infinite skills you could be developing. You'll stay focused, timely, and innovative in your niche area of specialty.

Finally, never worry that your ideal client is too specific. The more specific your ideal client character is, the faster your business will grow, the better outcomes you will help your clients achieve, and the more financially successful your practice will be. Just because your ideal client is a nurse in her thirties with a young child who likes triathlons and is struggling with anxiety and insomnia, doesn't mean that you won't attract working moms in their forties, male triathletes with anxiety, single doctors with insomnia, or other similar people. Just like you don't have to be a single coffee shop waitress to relate to Rachel from *Friends*, potential clients who relate to your ideal client character will see themselves in her and understand that you can help them.

6

COMMUNITY IS MEDICINE: THE SECRET TO GETTING MORE CLIENTS

Building community builds trust, and community is medicine. There are numerous studies that show that being a part of a community helps people to heal. For example, in a 2012 study published in *The Journal of Epidemiology and Community Health*, Hystad and Crapiano found that "...community-belonging showed a positive dose-response relationship with health-behavior change." An important strategy for improving trust, outcomes, and awareness of your niche practice is to build community among your clients and potential clients.

Creating communities of your potential ideal clients will position you as the problem solver for the group. While, ultimately, through the coaching process, your clients will individually solve their own health challenges, your role is as facilitator of the journey. Thus, for people to take the journey with you, they need to trust that you have the skills to lead them through this transformation.

Building community is also an effective marketing strategy for your practice. There are millions of health coaches, physical therapists, pilates instructors, nutritionists, massage therapists, yoga teachers, acupuncturists, and other health professionals. Why are some more successful than others? The successful practitioners are very clear about specifically who they work with, and the best coaches are very clear – even in their marketing messaging – that their process is collaborative with the client, and that the client will take a very active role. Plus, as we discussed in the last chapter, they are not trying to help everyone. The most successful coaches and practitioners are very clear about working with only the people that they are best equipped to help and most passionate about helping, and they stay focused on helping them solve one specific problem.

Speaking to everyone is a recipe for failure.

Building engaged communities of like-minded people who are all invested in helping themselves and each other to solve a specific problem brings clarity to your practice, helps you optimize your service, and allows you to fine tune your message. A deep understanding and connection with your ideal client combined with clear marketing messaging about the problem you help her to solve is the key to getting clients that you will enjoy working with and be successful at helping into your practice. Essentially all marketing tactics work, more or less. But you must find the marketing tactic or tactics that resonate most with your strengths that your ideal client is most interested in.

Thus, building communities of your ideal clients both online and offline is the secret sauce to building a support network to help your clients heal, and building excitement about your service among those who have yet to join your community of healing.

WHERE SHOULD I BUILD MY COMMUNITY?

Where to build your community starts with an assessment of your communication strengths and the locations where your ideal clients are likely already hanging out. First, assess how you best like to communicate. Are you obsessed with a certain social media platform, love its pace and content? For example, building your community on the Instagram platform could be great for you if you like visual content, like to use mobile posting strategies, and like consistently using the platform to connect with others who are also serving your ideal client. Conversely, if you like to write on in-depth topics, you might thrive on building a Medium platform, or a regular column in an online magazine. If you prefer live speaking, you might thrive on setting up a workshop series or speaking at large in-person or virtual events. The key is to enjoy the process because you have to do it consistently.

Ideally, there is an interactive component to your community. Your potential and active clients should be able to engage with you on the platform, ask questions, and share their experience from the "audience" – whether that is literally live and in-person, or via the comments section or chat box. Thus, not only should you enjoy regularly posting high quality content on the platform, but your ideal clients should be there. Ask yourself, does your ideal client "hang out" here anyway? Speaking in front of audiences online or offline is best when the audiences would be there anyway, saving you the work of getting them to the platform, event, or workshop in the first place.

WHAT DOES MY COMMUNITY WANT TO HEAR FROM ME?

The focus of all of your content should be about speaking directly to your ideal client about how to solve her number one problem. Each time you write a post, create a meme, film a video, or create a slide deck for an educational workshop, you should create that piece of content with only one goal in mind.

That goal is to help your ideal client solve her health problem and reach her health goal. When you keep your ideal client front and center in your mind when you're creating all content, and creating it just for her, it gets easier and easier to know what to say.

Exactly which questions to answer with your content will come from getting to know your client better. If you're already working with clients in your practice, start a journal and write down the questions that your ideal clients ask you in the clinic. If you're not working with clients yet, spend more time listening in supportive Facebook groups where your ideal client would hang out. If none exist, create a supportive Facebook group for your ideal client. Inevitably, questions will come up about what kind of content to create. Should I create deep-dive, detailed videos on complex topics, or thirty to ninety second "how to" videos? Should I write 3000 word, fully referenced blog posts, or 300 word "Top 5 Tips" articles? Should I tweet to my ideal client or write long, heartfelt stories on Facebook to my ideal client? The answer is always: how would she like to receive the information?

Consider this...if you're writing a message to good friend about a mutual friend who is getting over an illness, who you both know well, you will know whether she wants a 500word detailed email about your mutual friend's recovery or a quick text saying, "all is well, Jane is on her way home today."

Because you know your friend, you're clear about how she likes to receive content and in what format. This will become more and more true for your ideal client as you get to know her. This is why it's essential to interact with your ideal client in real life (online or offline) as much as possible.

Over the course of creating our endometriosis health coaching method, I have spoken individually to thousands of my ideal clients in phone consultations, live and interactive online workshops, and in group and individual coaching programs of various lengths and formats. I have spoken on large stages at endometriosis patient-centered events and on podcast interviews with hosts who have endometriosis themselves. The only way to really get to know your ideal client at a deep level is to talk with her, and that begins with listening to her.

If you don't know yet what kind of content your ideal client prefers, ask her. Does she like quick recipe guides or daily inspiration texts? Does she like to track her progress on apps or share it in a supportive community with update posts? Does she like to learn in a workshop setting or by reading an article or book? Your content strategy will be successful the more you connect with your ideal client in the way that she's already consuming content anyway. And the trick is to do it consistently, thus you have to enjoy the process too. Expect that it will take at least six months to three years of consistent content creation, content sharing, and weekly conversations with your ideal client in order to build up a full and thriving community.

HOW CAN I GET MY COMMUNITY MORE ENGAGED?

Perhaps you've been posting consistently for months or years, but it still feels like you're talking into the void. You're getting no replies in the comments, no questions on your live workshops, and no replies to your emails. That is very frustrating, and it's a signal that you're not resonating with your ideal client. If this is happening to you, consider the following issues that you'll need to address.

1. You're not clear and specific enough about who your ideal client is.
2. You're not speaking directly to your ideal client, you're not listening to her enough, and you're not encouraging her to respond.
3. You're not prompting your ideal client to engage with you on an emotional level.
4. You haven't told her that you can help her and offered her a clear call to action.

Let's review these common issues in detail. First, if you're not clear and specific enough about who your ideal client is and the challenge that she's trying to overcome, she won't recognize herself in your content and she won't know that you're talking to her. Second, if you don't speak clearly to her in language she can understand (not overly clinical language), then she won't know that you're talking to her. Third, if you're not asking her questions, appealing to her frustrations and hopes, and encouraging her to react, then she may be reading your content, but she won't feel called to respond. And, finally, she may be reading with and engaging with your content, but if you're not engaging with her (responding to every comment, every email reply, etc.), and regularly inviting her to a call with you to see if you can help her, she won't feel comfortable asking for your help.

The key is to stay in conversation. Be active on your chosen platform. Be open to questions. Challenge your community to take action, be engaging and encouraging. This is the mindset shift from clinician to coach. Remember that your ideal clients are *active* participants in their own healing journey. They are not standing passively by while you lecture them or tell them what to do. If you're struggling here, revisit Chapter 4 and keep practicing thinking in questions instead of thinking in recommendations. In addition, go back to Chapter 5, and keep refining your ideal client. It's a lifelong process to get to know her deeply and engage with her. Even in your marketing, your collaborative journey is beginning. This engagement during the marketing phase when she's not even your client yet and there is no pressure for her to be your client is the key to connecting with the best people to become your clients. They are ready to jump in, engage with the process, and take action right away.

Finally, your community should also be encouraged to support each other. Even before they are clients, people who participate on your platform and in your event audiences should be encouraged to and facilitated to connect with each other. They have a unique vantage point to cheer each other on and be supportive when one person in the community is struggling. Remember, "...community-belonging showed a positive dose-response relationship with health-behavior change" (Hystad and Crapiano, 2010). If you design any marketing materials, such as T-shirts or water bottles, to use to bring awareness to your practice, your clients and potential clients are more likely to wear, use, or display these materials if they represent not just you or your brand, but *their* place in your community. For example, if your coaching program is for new mothers to return to weekend road races without urinary leaking, what if your community, brand, and coaching program was called, "Strong Mother Runners?" The women in your community are more likely to wear a T-shirt emblazoned with "Strong Mother Runner" instead of "Jane's Postpartum Wellness Coaching." Make the community about your ideal client, not about you. Your role is to be the leader and facilitator of the community, but don't be afraid to let it expand to become larger than you.

7

FOUNDATIONAL NUTRITION IS THE KEY TO ROOT CAUSE HEALING

PART I: DIGESTION AND IMMUNE HEALTH

In the previous chapters, we discussed why and how specific health coaching communication tools and foundational marketing strategies are essential to the success of your practice. These skills are essential to optimal outcomes for your clients and for filling your practice in order for it to be financially successful. In this chapter and the following chapter, we're going to discuss the third essential pillar for building a successful health coaching practice, which is the ability to utilize foundational functional nutrition and lifestyle medicine tools to support optimal health.

Our motto at The Integrative Women's Health Institute is "Don't chase symptoms. Optimize systems."

In this chapter, we're going to start with the digestive and immune systems, which are key to resolving all common chronic women's health challenges. Nutrition is a key driver of health, and everyone eats. Thus, no matter what clinical background you came from, it's essential for you to commit to learning core nutrition skills. Supporting your clients to optimize their day-to-day nutrition habits makes a huge difference to their overall health.

In addition to food and supplements specifically, I challenge you to think even more holistically about the meaning of the word nutrition. From cellular health to population health, nutrition encompasses a broader view. Nutrition includes access to healing options such as safe spaces for walking, clean air, and vegetables, access to nature, safe work and home environments, art, pleasure, support at home, healthy relationships, and so on.

Functional nutrition is a systems approach. It's similar to Chinese medicine and Ayurvedic medicine in that it's a full system approach to optimizing the health of all of the physiologic systems, including digestive, immune, endocrine, musculoskeletal, cardiovascular, and so on. However, unlike in traditional medicine, this perspective does not divide the body into those systems as being separate from one another. We understand in systems medicine that the nervous system is not separate from the cardiovascular system, musculoskeletal system, or immune system. Thus, when taking a functional nutrition approach, we often talk about the connections and interfaces between these systems as well. From a practical standpoint, we'll take a system by system approach in order to make it easier to learn how to prioritize healing strategies and actions. For example, your client can't use nutrient supplements or food to support healing of the nervous system effectively if the digestive system is compromised and can't absorb nutrients well.

One of the most powerful questions you can ask your clients as you begin your work with them is, "When did you feel the most well?" If they can remember a time when they felt well, which is not always possible, then there is a place to begin to help them regain that sense of health and wellbeing. What did they eat when they felt most well? Who was in their support network? What were they doing day-to-day? Did they have an exercise or mindfulness practice? What habits did they have around sleep?

When it comes to optimizing digestion we will take a tip to tail, or brain to anus if you will, approach. We don't consider the digestive system in isolation. We'll consider your client's digestion in the context of her overall life and health history. The health timeline is a valuable tool to see when her symptoms really began, flared, or were exacerbated.

If you ask your clients to document their health starting as early as preconception, including how healthy their parents were, you will often notice some interesting patterns.

For example, perhaps your client remembers that she started experiencing digestive problems back in sixth grade when her parents got divorced and she had to move. Perhaps she also developed anxiety around that time. Then, in college, she had a serious sports injury, had to stop training, and developed an eating disorder. Then, earlier this year she struggled with chronic UTIs and was prescribed five rounds of antibiotics. Now, in her late twenties, she's seeing you for chronic pain. Did this pain come out of nowhere? Or is it a longer term cumulative response to the breakdown in her support network, adverse childhood experiences, poor nutrition, stress, medication effects, lack of ability to exercise, toxic exposures, and so on? Most of the time, when people present to you for health coaching, their health challenge didn't just come out of nowhere, it is usually related to years or decades of cumulative life and health events. Our role as clinicians with a coaching mindset is to help our clients to see how their past is affecting their health, consider when they felt most healthy, and look for adaptive health behaviors that they can start to consistently implement along their healing journey.

A FOCUS ON OPTIMIZING HEALTH, NOT CURING DISEASE

In today's health landscape, many issues are chronic and overlapping. So, as we consider the digestive and immune systems, consider that your client may have any number of diagnoses, but what's important in our coaching perspective is to start with what's working well and build on that. In addition, remember that your role is to hold space for your client to define what being well means to her. The clearer that her vision becomes through the coaching process, and the more she takes action towards her goals along the way, the easier it will be for her to take the daily health behavior steps necessary to live into her vision.

START WITH DIGESTION

There are three things to consider when it comes to digestion. What food is your client eating, what supplements is she taking, and how well is the digestive system functioning? Thus, not only are most of our clients not eating enough nutrient dense food and too much processed food, but most people also have digestive challenges that make it difficult for them to absorb the nutrients that they are eating. Nutrient deficiencies are extremely common. Even high level collegiate athletes are commonly nutrient deficient. Thus, what your client eats is very important.

Fortunately, there are a wide range of healthy diets. Healthy diets span from vegan to Mediterranean to ketogenic. There is not one perfect diet. The most optimal diet for any given client depends on their genetics, activity levels, food sensitivities, other health issues, food preferences, ethical preferences, and access to foods. To determine which food plan is best for your ideal client, start by having her fill out a three-day food journal.

With a coaching mindset, we can then help her to identify and eat more of the foods that help her to feel more energized, sleep better, and have better digestive function. Often your clients have some idea of what foods feel best for them. Not always, and that's a more complex topic outside of the scope of this book. Sometimes your clients will have significant food intolerances, confusion about what foods to eat based on information overwhelm, and/or eating disorders. As a health coach, while your knowledge of nourishing eating and optimal digestive function is important, there will be an upper limit to your understanding. Thus, it's often going to be important for you to also help your client find the right nutrition professional for her team. One of the most important roles of a health coach is to support your client in building a supportive health team for herself. Each client's team will be different but may include a nutrition professional, a physical therapist, a fitness professional, primary care physician, gynecologist or other specialist, mental health professional, and so on.

Remember that the food journal is Step 1 for helping your client connect to her own nutrition wisdom. Nearly all of your clients will have some understanding of which foods feel most supportive for their health. You can try this yourself. Fill out a three-day food journal (see the bonus materials at http://clinic2coach.com/). Then, start with a simple screening to be sure that your foundational nutrition needs are being met.

- Are you eating eight to ten servings of vegetables per day?
- Are you eating one to two servings of fruit per day?
- Are you eating approximately 0.8g to 2g per kg of body weight of clean protein each day?
- Are you eating approximately 30 percent of each meal in healthy fats, such as olive oil, avocado, or nuts and seeds?
- Are you drinking sixty to one hundred ounces per day of filtered or mineral water daily?

As you can already tell, I'm not a fan of

prescribing a diet based on a disease label, but there is some data supporting certain dietary perspectives for certain populations, and certain diagnoses that are useful to explore for your specific ideal client community. From that perspective, are ketogenic diets really the opposite of vegan diets? Why do both raw vegan diets and ketogenic diets help with pain? These can both be highly nutrient dense diets or they could be all vegan cookies or bacon. The key is not just the macronutrient composition, but also the nutrient density and quality of the food plan.

This is where, I believe, most of our perspective on nutrition is just wrong. In the Western world, nutrition education is all about restriction of the "fun" foods instead of indulging in nourishing and delicious foods. If we keep our focus on digestive health, eating low inflammatory foods that are nutrient rich can be delicious! From a coaching mindset and behavior change standpoint, doesn't it make sense to support people in eating a more delicious, nutrient-dense diet rather than to encourage "willpower" to restrict the diet? Nutrient-dense diets can be delicious. Starting the conversation there is far more likely to support our clients towards long term healthy behaviors.

Once you assess the diet with the three-day food journal, consider the most common foods that she's eating that contribute to inflammation. Commonly eaten inflammatory foods include processed and fried foods, sugar, dairy, gluten, and soy. There are other foods that can be inflammatory for different people at different times, but these are the most common, so we'll start there. In addition to foods being inflammatory, the environment and lifestyle of your client can also be inflammatory. Perhaps your client has been exposed to heavy metals or other environmental toxins. Perhaps she's under a lot of financial stress or is living in an abusive relationship. Maybe she's living with an underlying chronic infection. When we take a broad and integrative perspective, it's easier to see that food is not always the core problem.

In addition to considering her diet, consider how your client is eating. Is your client relaxed and eating with pleasure, or is she eating on the run? Is she afraid that eating will trigger her symptoms or struggling with body image issues? Is she stressed out by the people she's sitting down to eat with? Optimal digestion is dependent on eating in a relaxed environment with healthy levels of digestive juices flowing, a calm nervous system, and healthy hormone levels.

Start with chewing. This is huge. The evidence shows that chewing forty times per bite is ideal. Now to be fair, this study was done using almonds, so that's a pretty hard food; but still, notice next time how many times you chew any one bite before you swallow. Three? One? Ten? During your next meal, slow down, and observe how well you chew or how quickly you tend to rush through your meal. Is it challenging for you to slow down and chew?

The digestive process starts with chewing. Then food moves to the stomach. There, adequate stomach acid is key, especially for the digestion of proteins. Low stomach acid levels are common for people with chronic fatigue or chronic pain conditions since it takes so much physiologic energy, or ATP, to produce stomach acid. Plus, long term use of acid-reducing medications such as proton pump inhibitors is common, despite the fact that these medications were designed for short term use, ideally sixteen weeks or less. I have worked with clients who have been on acid lowering medications for decades! Imagine how difficult it is for their bodies to absorb essential amino acids!

There are a number of ways to test for low stomach acid, otherwise known as hypochlorhydria. In medical offices, a test called The Heidelberg Test sends a pill-sized pH sensor into the stomach to measure the stomach acid directly. This works well and is well supported by over 150 clinical studies. However, it's challenging and can be impractical. Clinically, I support healthy stomach acid using what's known as The Betaine HCL Challenge. Start with one capsule of Betaine HCL at the beginning of the heaviest protein meal. Some supplements also contain pepsin, which is an enzyme that is activated by stomach acid to allow you to more easily digest protein. You can also use a separate digestive enzyme supplement with a variety of enzymes to support the digestion of protein, fats, and carbohydrates.

When you've taken one capsule of the Betaine HCL supplement at the beginning of your heaviest protein meal, notice how you feel. If you notice nothing or that your digestion feels better, continue taking one capsule at the beginning of your heaviest protein meal for the rest of the week. If you notice any symptoms of heartburn, such as burning in your chest, arms, or back, or other signs of indigestion, stop using the Betaine HCL supplement.

If all feels well, you feel improved digestion, or you don't notice any change in your digestion, then, the next week, increase the dose to two capsules with your heaviest protein meal each day. Continue for another week, then increase the dose to three capsules at the beginning of your heaviest protein meal each day.

If you start to feel symptoms of heartburn or indigestion at any dose (for example, with three capsules) reduce the dose back to the previous beneficial dose (for example, reduce the dose down from three to two capsules where you didn't feel any uncomfortable symptoms, just better digestion). Rarely, it can take high doses of Betaine HCL before digestion begins to improve. However, I highly recommend working with your functional nutritionist or physician to optimize your dose. Don't try to do this on your own. There are some risks to adding Betaine HCL to your nutrition plan. This supplemental acid can contribute to ulcers. Do not do this test if you have a history of ulcers or any inflammatory bowel disease.

As the food then moves along the digestive tract, the next step is further digestion by digestive enzymes. How do we test for healthy digestive enzyme levels? Fortunately, stool testing can measure pancreatic elastase levels. The optimal level of pancreatic elastase is 400 micrograms per gram. If the levels are lower, then supplemental pancreatic elastase is needed. There are specific enzyme supplements that can also be required if they are genetically lacking, such as Diamine oxidase (DAO), which breaks down histamine. Culinary herbs and spices also support the release of healthy digestive enzymes. Adding herbs and spices such as oregano, turmeric, mint, dill, fennel, ginger, garlic and more to enhance the flavor of food also supports ease of digestion of food.

THE SMALL INTESTINE: THE INTERFACE BETWEEN THE DIGESTIVE AND IMMUNE SYSTEMS

Most nutrients are absorbed in the small intestine, and two common issues often disrupt nutrient absorption at the lining of the small interesting. However, for many people, the health of the lining of the small intestine is compromised. The digestive lining is easily irritated by stress, by food that is not well broken down (due to lack of chewing and/ or low digestive juices), by processed foods, sugar and other inflammatory foods, and the other causes of inflammation that we discussed above. Medications such as NSAIDs and antibiotics can also disrupt the delicate environment of the small intestine and lining of the small intestine.

The lining of the small intestine is one key interface between the digestive and immune systems. Don't forget that the lining of the digestive tract is like an "inner skin." Food comes into the digestive tract from the outside world. Thus, it's not sterile. Chewing and stomach acid are designed to kill off some of the microbes that come into our bodies on our food, but if those systems are compromised, the microbes can invade. In that case, when there are challenges with the lining of the small intestine where the food should be absorbed but microbes and other toxins kept out, the immune system can be activated, increasing inflammation and risk of autoimmune attacks. The loss of the protective function of the small intestinal barrier and/or imbalances or overgrowths in the bacteria that are supposed to augment that barrier can set your client up for immune system breakdown.

The immune system is designed to be diligent to be able to kill off invaders that hitch a ride on our food and try to infect us. But the immune system also has to stay in balance. It should not be in "attack mode" all of the time. There needs to be tolerance to the outside world. We should not be over reactive to normal environmental molecules, such as foods, dust, pollen, and pets. Our bodies should be able to turn off the inflammatory action of the immune system using functioning regulatory T cells. If inflammation becomes chronic, then lifestyle diseases occur such as diabetes, cardiovascular disease, stroke, and heart attacks. The goal is for the immune system to mount a healthy immune response to bacterial pathogens and viruses and to keep cancer in check. But the immune system also must be kept in check to tolerate human cells and non-pathogenic molecules like pollen. It's a delicate balance between fighting invaders and then resolving the inflammation and tolerating our own cells and our environment. Excessive inflammation actually suppresses the immune system because when the system is always on, it's not able to target invaders efficiently.

NOURISHMENT THAT OPTIMIZES DIGESTION AND SUPPORTS HEALTHY IMMUNE FUNCTION

The good news is that there are many delicious and enjoyable ways to quiet inflammation and enhance both digestion and immune function. Anti-inflammatory nutrients are delicious and available. To name just a few… turmeric in curry powder, green tea, gamma linolenic acid (GLA) a fatty acid found in breast milk, fish oil, rosemary, vitamin D from sun exposure, cinnamon, blueberries, and many more. Don't forget non-food nourishment. Spending time in nature, pleasure, and laughter release oxytocin, an anti-inflammatory hormone.

THE GUT MICROBIOME

In addition to our own digestive function, both our digestive and immune systems are supported by a healthy balance of microbes in the intestines, with especially large numbers in the colon.

What are some factors that disturb a healthy microbiome? Most commonly, antibiotics. For many of your clients, look at their timelines for exposures to antibiotics (often many exposures) through their lifetimes. What can be done to measure the health of the colon microbiome? Clinically, I utilize stool testing. Stool testing has its limitations because we don't know what the ideal composition of the gut microbiome should be. Generally, using these tests, your client's stool will be compared to stool samples from young adults with no functional limitations, significant symptoms, or diagnoses. That doesn't guarantee that the comparative ranges are optimal, but it's the best approximation that we have for now.

If the gut microbiome is out of optimal balance, if there are signs of inflammation or low immune resilience – such as low mucosal SIgA in the lining of the small intestine – lead with a coaching mindset. Think, "How should we restore balance?" Remember to start by asking your client about when her digestion and immune resilience felt best. From the very beginning, support your client to tune into her intuition and take cues from her physical signals. Perhaps she'll say, "My digestion felt best when I was eating a lot of salads," or "My digestion felt best when I was eating mostly light soups." Perhaps she'll be aware of better bowel movements when she ate more fermented foods or easier digestion when she was better hydrated. Perhaps she feels that stress or poor sleep impacts her digestion and immune resilience. Start with what she already knows can be supportive of her health, and coach her to take those health-enhancing actions consistently.

In general, healthy digestion and immune function loves routine. We'll talk more about the circadian rhythm in the next chapter. And know that regular bowel movements are encouraged by a consistent bowel schedule and morning routine.

Health optimization starts in the gut. Supporting your client to define for herself and enjoy an anti-inflammatory diet and lifestyle goes a long way towards optimizing health from the root. An anti-inflammatory diet alone reduces the risk of all-cause mortality by 18 percent! (Kaluza, et al, 2019) As the digestive and immune systems become more resilient, it's easier to optimize the health of all of the other systems because your client can finally absorb the nutrients that she needs to fully heal.

References:

Kaluza, J., Håkansson, N., Harris, H. R., Orsini, N., Michaëlsson, K., & Wolk, A. (2019). Influence of anti-inflammatory diet and smoking on mortality and survival in men and women: two prospective cohort studies. *Journal of internal medicine*, 285(1), 75–91. https://doi.org/10.1111/joim.12823

FOUNDATIONAL NUTRITION IS THE KEY TO ROOT CAUSE HEALING

PART 2: NEUROENDOCRINE HEALTH

"It's not brain surgery."

In modern medicine, we often believe that for complex systems such as the nervous and endocrine systems, symptom healing has to be complicated and expensive. Our clinical training is long, detailed, complex, and expensive, and I believe that our training sets us up to start with the most complex interventions before fully utilizing highly effective, simpler, foundational lifestyle and intuitive health behaviors first. I can't tell you the number of times in my coaching practice for women with endometriosis and complex pelvic pain conditions that I've seen clients who have "failed treatment" at renowned institutions like The Mayo Clinic, or who have been prescribed twenty-five supplements by famous functional medicine doctors, but who have not been shown how to consistently implement the foundational lifestyle medicine actions that are essential to their healing.

Of course, complex interventional medicine is important at times. And sometimes, we start with the most complex diagnostic interventions to rule out serious conditions that are more likely to be resolved the sooner we take action. For example, if a woman presents to her gynecologist with pelvic pain, ruling out ovarian cancer, an unlikely possibility, with expensive imaging could literally save her life. But approximately 21,000 people are diagnosed with ovarian cancer each year in the United States, while over eleven million women each year struggle with other causes of pelvic pain that can be significantly improved with lifestyle medicine strategies. Endometriosis is perhaps a special case because early, skilled surgical consultation is so important. Early surgical consultation leads to better outcomes, especially in concert with pre- and post-operative nutrition, physical therapy, and lifestyle medicine interventions. But the bottom line is that the vast majority of our most common challenges, including chronic pain, chronic fatigue, dementia, obesity, metabolic syndrome, cardiovascular disease, and even many infectious diseases benefit far more from foundational, consistent healthy lifestyle behaviors than any expensive medications or surgeries

The healthcare transformation will be led by the clinicians who adopt a coaching mindset of supporting the patient to take an active, collaborative leadership role in her care and who are willing to put in the consistent effort to support their clients to implement foundational daily health behaviors. It's time to shift the paradigm, and even for seemingly complex symptoms including pain and fatigue, **don't skip the foundation**.

WHAT IS "THE FOUNDATION" OF HEALTH BEHAVIORS?

Everything begins in the brain for both nervous system-related symptoms and hormone health. Because all of the hormonal axes - adrenal (stress), thyroid (metabolism), and reproductive - begin with signaling from the hypothalamus, understand that all hormone health conditions start in the brain. So, what are the foundational, daily health actions that are essential to brain health?

- Nutrient absorption
- Blood sugar stability
- Sleep
- Stress resilience
- Energy

NUTRIENT ABSORPTION AND BLOOD SUGAR STABILITY

As a prerequisite for healthy nutrient absorption, review the last chapter. Digestive function is key to the brain's ability to absorb nutrients. The brain is primarily fueled by a steady stream of glucose, unlike the rest of the body, which can run on stored glycogen in the liver. The brain does have a small amount of glycogen stored in the astrocytes, but it's just enough to stave off severe hypoglycemic or anemic emergencies. In some cases, the brain can run on ketones. But, in most cases, a stable flow of glucose is key to brain nourishment.

Blood sugar balance is a daily lifestyle habit. The key to balancing blood sugar is to, counterintuitively, eat much less sugar and avoid alcohol. Instead, when your clients eat every six hours, sometimes more often at first, a meal of high-quality protein, healthy fat, and fiber (mostly vegetables) over the course of a few days to a few months, their blood sugar stability will be dramatically improved. It's that simple. By making this one change, chronic pain, fatigue, chronic infections, risk of getting colds, flus, and other viruses, weight loss resistance, and more can be dramatically improved. Your client's sleep will improve, her daily energy will improve, and her brain fog will lift.

This sounds like miracle medicine! Why is everyone not doing this? It's *so simple*!

Yes, but...most people are both physically and emotionally addicted to sugar and/or alcohol. Plus, sweetened, highly processed carbohydrate foods are often less expensive, faster and easier to prepare, and more readily available.

How can you screen your client to see if she's struggling with blood sugar instability? Following is the analogy I use to screen my patients. Imagine that today, I said to you, "I'm going to give you a free ticket to Paris (you live in New York.) That's a ten-plus-hour journey from your apartment in New York to landing in your hotel room in Paris. But here's the catch, you may not eat anything from the moment you leave your apartment until you arrive in your hotel room in Paris. If you're feeling a little panicked by just reading that, then you likely have blood sugar instability."

I used to be the same way. When I worked at a major teaching hospital as an inpatient physical therapist, I used to wear a lab coat. It was part of my uniform, but it wasn't required. I wore the lab coat because I was away from my desk all day running around the hospital working with patients. The lab coat had pockets. I needed those pockets so I could stash protein bars or other snacks to carry with me. I couldn't go four hours, never mind ten, waiting for my lunch break to eat. If I did, I would get jittery, anxious, and shaky. These are all signs of reactive hypoglycemia. Reactive hypoglycemia is the most common initial symptom of blood sugar instability, later it can progress to other metabolic issues such as prediabetes, polycystic ovarian syndrome (PCOS), thyroid issues, adrenal dysregulation, and diabetes.

Reactive hypoglycemia is the response to excessive intake of sugar, alcohol, and/or processed carbohydrates (like breads or pastas). In women, it's likely to be worse in the luteal phase of the menstrual cycle or menopause, when the insulin sensitivity effects of estrogen are reduced. First, blood sugar is elevated (by eating a highly processed, sweetened meal or snack), then insulin jumps in to save your life and shuttle the sugar into the cells. Because that is an emergency situation that your insulin is reacting to, it tends to overreact. A couple of hours after this high sugar meal, your blood sugar will crash due to the over response of excessive insulin secretion, prompting a reaction from the hormone cortisol to elevate the blood sugar. This process is known as the blood sugar roller coaster. It's a very damaging ride to brain and endocrine health.

When blood sugar is unstable, your client will present with symptoms of anxiety, shakiness, sugar cravings, sleep disturbances (when this process happens in the middle of the night waking her up), hormonal symptoms like period pain, irregular periods, hot flashes, abdominal fat gain, brain fog, and memory loss. Usually treating these symptoms starts with complex interventions that can come with serious side effects like progesterone creams, sleep medications, pain medications, caffeine, birth control pills, and serotonin reuptake inhibitors. Sometimes these complex interventions might be necessary. But first, in our transformational model of healthcare, we'll coach our clients to bring awareness to the possibility that her blood sugar is unstable. If it is, we'll support her to make the daily nutrition and lifestyle changes needed to balance her blood sugar. Then, most of the time, when blood sugar balancing lifestyle strategies are used, none of these other interventions will be necessary.

In addition to optimizing blood sugar stability, the brain needs nourishment. We have high levels of iron deficiency, which reduces oxygenation to the brain. We have stomach acid deficiency and lack of quality protein intake, which limits the flow of amino acids to the brain. Amino acids are the building blocks of all of the brain's neurotransmitters. Plus, inflammation related to low intake and absorption of antioxidants limits brain function.

Thus, as I mentioned in the previous chapter, we have to focus our nutrition interventions on supporting people to ADD nourishment, not restrict their diets. Eating quality proteins, fats, and vegetables at each meal supports foundational nervous system function, which is the cornerstone of hormonal health at all levels.

SLEEP AND STRESS RESILIENCE

The importance of quality, consistent sleep cannot be overstated. And yet, with poor daily lifestyle habits and significant challenges with social determinants of health, such as excessive screen time, lack of safe living spaces, limited exposure to nature, financial stress, and lack of community, achieving optimal sleep is nearly impossible.

Interestingly, the brain and the bowels (a key indicator of digestive health) both thrive on routine. Yet, how many of our clients are burning the candle at both ends, not implementing consistent morning or evening routines, and struggling with energy crashes on a daily basis?

I mentioned above that the "blood sugar rollercoaster" will certainly impact sleep, and following are several other strategies that are simple, foundational factors that impact sleep.

Screen your clients for the following: Do they:

- Turn off all blue light devices (cell phones, laptops, televisions, etc.) by eight p.m.?
- Get at least fifteen minutes of daylight exposure each day (without sunglasses)?
- Sleep in a dark/quiet/cool room?

- Have a comfortable/supportive mattress/pillow?
- Have a bedtime routine?
- Avoid caffeine (or limit it to before noon)?
- Only use their bed for sex, light reading, or sleep?

These foundational sleep strategies combined with a daily commitment to keeping blood sugar optimized will significantly improve sleep quality.

It's also important to consider the two rhythms of sleep: the circadian rhythm and the adenosine rhythm. The circadian is your daylight and night rhythm. When it gets dark outside, stress hormone (cortisol) levels should be at their lowest levels of the day. Darkness stimulates the release of melatonin, stimulating quality sleep. If cortisol levels are high, cortisol will inhibit the release of melatonin. The amino acid tryptophan (remember the importance of protein intake and absorption) is an important building block of serotonin, and melatonin is derived from serotonin (Masters, et al., 2014). Regularly receiving therapeutic massage therapy and optimal magnesium levels are other factors that support healthy melatonin levels (Cao, et al., 2018 & Ferber, et al, 2002).

The second sleep rhythm, the adenosine rhythm, is related to the fact that adenosine receptors play an important role in inducing sleep and optimizing the sleep-wake cycle. Adenosine is the by-product of adenosine triphosphate (ATP) breakdown. ATP is essentially cellular energy. Thus, activity during the day – including exercise, movement, and mental acuity and activity – will promote sleep. Caffeine blocks the adenosine receptor. This is why limiting or eliminating caffeine production is also sleep promoting.

Therefore, a daily focus on (ideally outdoor) movement and activity, attention to light and dark rhythms, and elimination of sugar, alcohol, and caffeine are simple, foundational habits that can result in significant improvements in sleep duration and quality. Most people are not doing these foundational things consistently over the long term. That's where health coaching comes in. Why aren't people doing these basic things, and instead reaching for sleep medications, or pinning their hopes on miracle supplements? Why? Because consistently doing these things is counter to the pressures of modern life. Our clients are busy, highly stressed, addicted to caffeine and their screens, and are dependent on things that are detrimental to their sleep quality to survive their high stress lifestyles.

Sleep and stress optimization can begin with one simple intervention, the "sleepcation." This is a tool that I learned from Dr. Alan Christianson in his book, *The Adrenal Reset Diet*. This sleep reset is to simply spend three consecutive days without any screens simply relaxing, being in nature, and sleeping as much as your body wants to. A similarly effective reset is camping for three nights. Camping for just three nights, again without screens, has been shown to rapidly reset circadian timing via the effect of natural light exposure (Stothard, et al., 2017).

Of course, sleep is also affected by chronic stressors. In my experience, 99 percent of all core stressors involve three things:

- Stress surrounding a close relationship (marital strain, sick child, difficulty with one's boss)
- Grief
- Work or financial stress

The most common stressors in The United States according to Harvard University's School of Public Health are:

- Too many responsibilities
- Problems with finances
- Work problems
- Health problems
- Health problems of an immediate family member
- Problems with family members
- Being unhappy with the way you look

As you can see, most of these challenges are behavioral or social, not biochemical. Thus, if we don't use coaching interventions to address the underlying social and behavioral problems that people struggle with, all of the supplement and medication recommendations in the world will not be very effective. People have choices about how to deal with their stressors, but often the stress is so ubiquitous that they are not even aware of their stressors and the fact that strategies exist to minimize their stressors. This is what's possible if clinical healthcare transforms to leading with a coaching model. If instead of recommending massage, Ambien, or lavender oil as quick fixes for sleep, we start to focus on why people aren't sleeping well (and all of the other consequences of the significant burden of stress), we can get to the root of the many health problems that stem from poor sleep and chronic stress.

If we take a coaching and integrative healing perspective, and go beyond fixing sleep symptoms and reducing stressors to helping our clients bathe their nervous systems daily in signals of safety, this can take healing even deeper. I learned the concepts of DIMs (Signals of "Danger in My Body") and SIMs (Signals of "Safety in My Body") from Dr. Lorimer Moseley and Dr. David Butler in their book, *The Explain Pain Handbook Protectometer.* Clinical healthcare does not emphasize feeling well or a focus on when we feel well. About a decade ago, I stopped asking my chronic pain clients to constantly focus on tracking and telling me their pain levels, and instead to start keeping a small journal and write down anytime they feel a little better or notice a few minutes without pain. When they noticed small moments of feeling well or even just a bit better, I instructed them to write down what was going on at the time. Answering questions like... What were you wearing? What were you eating or drinking? Who were you with? What were you thinking about? How were you feeling? This was such an important shift in my clients pain relief and recovery that I began to screen for and track pleasure and wellness instead of pain.

Following are the questions I ask to screen for pleasure. Do you:

- Know at least three people, things, or situations that bring you pleasure?
- Enjoy fun daily? Weekly?
- Laugh? Daily? Weekly?

Surround yourself with at least two people who you just adore at least weekly (might be via phone or video conference)?

Shifting our focus from sickness to health is another important transformation in mindset from thinking like a clinician to thinking like a coach. As you're probably starting to see, transforming hundreds of thousands of healthcare professions from thinking like a clinician – looking for problems to "fix," – to thinking like a coach – looking for systems to optimize – is how we will collectively transform healthcare away from its dangerous focus on sick-care.

ENERGY

Finally, I want to discuss the important foundational health behaviors that are key to energy and mitochondrial function. This attention to daily energy enhancing habits is valuable for overcoming our epidemic of fatigue and distraction. My perspective on energy optimization comes from looking at mitochondrial health and lowering environmental toxin load.

Starting with screening for environmental toxins, these are the questions I ask my clients.

Do you:

- Consider the environmental toxin load of your shampoos, skincare, and cosmetics?
- Limit your exposure to plastic – flip flops, food containers, water bottles?
- Drink filtered water?
- Know your region's air quality?

- Have air filtering plants or air filters in your home and office?
- Consider your electromagnetic field (EMF) exposure?
- Spend at least thirty minutes per day in nature?
- Consciously address toxic relationships?
- Bring awareness to and actively work on limiting your toxic thoughts?
- Participate in psychosocial therapies to heal past traumas?

As you can see, there are toxins everywhere. They are in our environment, our homes, our relationships, and even our thoughts. Initially, it's important to simply bring attention to these daily strains on your client's energy. Imagine that every one of your clients is carrying a backpack filled with their toxic energy drains. Everyone will always have a backpack as long as they are alive, but using the coaching process and implementing behavioral strategies to address some of these issues can significantly lighten the weight of each client's backpack and build communities of supportive people to carry their backpacks for them sometimes.

On the flip side, mitochondrial function can also be actively enhanced using a variety of behavioral and integrative approaches. First of all, what are the mitochondria? As you might remember from Biology 101, the mitochondria are the powerhouses of every cell. Thus, biochemically, they are key to energy! For the mitochondria to function optimally, they must also be nourished. Mitochondrial function declines in an environment of oxidative stress. Fortunately, antioxidants are the antidote to oxidative stress. Additionally, a healthy and diverse population of gut microbes communicates directly with the mitochondria enhancing their health. Specific behavioral strategies that support mitochondrial function are as follows:

- Eating diets rich in nutrients that reduce oxidative stress, including vitamins A, C, and E, N-acetyl-cysteine, glutathione, and alpha lipoic acid
- Quitting smoking
- Exercising regularly
- Eating fiber and probiotic foods

Again, there is no silver bullet energy drink, high dose supplement, or medication that delivers focused energy, but there are daily lifestyle factors that combine to support healthy energy levels. With good mitochondrial function, people feel so much better. Brain fog and mild memory loss are reduced, pain is reduced, fatigue is reduced, and productivity is enhanced. An energized life is a healthier and more enjoyable life!

References:

Cao, Y., Zhen, S., Taylor, A. W., Appleton, S., Atlantis, E., & Shi, Z. (2018). Magnesium Intake and Sleep Disorder Symptoms: Findings from the Jiangsu Nutrition Study of Chinese Adults at Five-Year Follow-Up. Nutrients, 10 (10), 1354. https://doi.org/10.3390/nu10101354

Ferber, S. G., Laudon, M., Kuint, J., Weller, A., & Zisapel, N. (2002). Massage therapy by mothers enhances the adjustment of circadian rhythms to the nocturnal period in full-term infants. Journal of developmental and behavioral pediatrics : JDBP, 23 (6), 410–415. https://doi.org/10.1097/00004703-200212000-00003

Masters, A., Pandi-Perumal, S. R., Seixas, A., Girardin, J. L., & McFarlane, S. I. (2014). Melatonin, the Hormone of Darkness: From Sleep Promotion to Ebola Treatment. Brain disorders & therapy, 4 (1), 1000151. https://doi.org/10.4172/2168-975X.1000151

Stothard, E. R., McHill, A. W., Depner, C. M., Birks, B. R., Moehlman, T. M., Ritchie, H. K., Guzzetti, J. R., Chinoy, E. D., LeBourgeois, M. K., Axelsson, J., & Wright, K. P., Jr (2017). Circadian Entrainment to the Natural Light-Dark Cycle across Seasons and the Weekend. Current biology : CB, 27 (4), 508–513. https://doi.org/10.1016/j.cub.2016.12.041

9

WHY MOST HEALTHCARE PROFESSIONALS ARE AFRAID TO COACH

In the previous chapters, you learned the steps to make a successful transformation from a clinician to a coaching mindset, and you learned how to build a financially successful health coaching practice from the ground up. Unfortunately, most people, even with this knowledge, don't run out and build their ideal health coaching practice.

Why?

Most healers don't make the transition from clinician to creating their own successful health coaching practice for three reasons: lack of trust, fear, and the inability to be decisive.

LACK OF TRUST

Coming from a clinically trained background myself, I understand how hard it can be to trust that your client knows her next best step in her healing journey. While it's true that sometimes she doesn't know what to do next, very often she does. This was surprising for me to experience with my clients since my clinical training emphasized the importance of expertise, clinical decision-making, pattern recognition, and my role in telling my clients what to do for them to heal. I was surprised to discover that often my clients know what to do, they just aren't doing it (for many reasons that the coaching process can address).

In fact, often I would tell clients – using my deep clinical expertise – exactly what they would need to do to relieve their symptoms, and they still wouldn't do it. Let me share a story…

Many years ago, when I was still a practicing pelvic physical therapist full time in an outpatient clinic, one of my patients presented me with a very clear bladder diary. We used bladder diaries to help look for food or hydration triggers for urinary incontinence in the pelvic physical therapy clinic. This patient had the clearest diary I had ever seen. The diary clearly showed both of us that the only time she would leak urine is when she would drink Diet Dr. Pepper. As soon as I saw this, I was thrilled. Problem solved! I am such a genius, this woman's years of struggle with incontinence could be over today!

Well, it could have been over that day, except…

she was completely unwilling to give up Diet Dr. Pepper. No way. She literally said to me, "If I have to choose between Diet Dr. Pepper and peeing on myself for the rest of my life, I will choose to pee on myself." What?! I was shocked. But, this is a great example of why telling people what they "should" do for their health, doesn't work. I worked with her before I was very skilled in health coaching, but I did use some health coaching skills to negotiate with her. We eventually agreed that she would drink just one Diet Dr. Pepper in the morning, when she was still home, deal with her leaks at home, and then go about her day. And, if she was going to drink one later in the day, she would be prepared with a pad. We did other things to address her overall pelvic strength and health, but eliminating the Diet Dr. Pepper was the final key to her leaking pattern.

Bottom line is, we have to *trust* that our clients know the best next step in their healing journeys, they just aren't taking those steps because of a myriad of internal and external barriers to change. Until those are addressed, they can get all of the recommendations in the world that could literally save their lives or solve their primary health problem, and they won't do them.

Want other examples? Consider that...

- Smoking: 14 percent of American adults

still smoke, yet everyone knows that smoking is bad for their health.

- Seatbelts: 14 percent of American adults refuse to wear seatbelts, yet everyone knows that seatbelts save lives in auto accidents.
- Binge drinking: 16 percent of American adults binge drink alcohol, yet everyone knows that binge drinking is bad for their health.
- I could go on and on. Knowing what to do is not the same as doing it when it comes to health behaviors. And, when your clients truly get stuck and don't know what to do yet, you can shift gears to clinical and educator modes and support them in figuring out their next steps.

FEAR

It's scary to be on the cutting edge. The healthcare system transformation is scary. We don't know what's going to be built next. It's hard to imagine what the system will look like in the future. It can feel risky to stick our necks out and lead this revolution, but we must. If the most committed, compassionate, and skilled healers don't take this transformation by the reins, someone else will… someone more concerned with profits over patients, someone more concerned with efficiency than care, someone less creative, caring, or innovative than you. We need you! It's time for you to step up and lead!

What are some of the specific fears that our Integrative Women's Health Institute Health Coaching students and graduates overcome when they are building their successful practices?

- Fear of asking for help.
- Fear of being criticized by colleagues, family, friends, or others.
- Fear of giving up control of the healing process and trusting their clients more.
- Fear of building a solid business with the help of legal, financial, accounting, or insurance experts.
- Fear of making a mistake.
- Fear of ruffling the feathers of their licensing boards.
- Fear of marketing.
- Fear of sales.
- Fear of investing in their businesses until they are already making money.

The most common fear that my students must overcome is fear of "doing this wrong." I am often asked, "Can I coach people with my clinical license?" "What certifications do I need?" "Is this legal?" The interesting thing about these questions is that they hinge on another key fear, the fear of asking for help. I am not an attorney. I can't answer any of these questions for them. But every business owner should be working with skilled professionals in the areas of legal, financial, accounting, and insurance. If you don't have people with these skills on speed dial, you haven't decided to build a real business. Nearly everything you'll want to do with your coaching practice is likely legal or in a legal gray area. You probably don't want to do anything dangerous, unethical, or harmful. I'm sure you've read this far in this book because you really want to help people in a way that's more effective and sustainable for both them and you. Thus, it's likely that all you'll need to do to cover your bases is to ask for professional advice and put the appropriate documents and paperwork in place. But most clinicians really struggle with asking for this kind of help. It's as if you should also be an expert in all of these things. It's okay – in fact, it's expected that you're not an expert in business financing, accounting, insurance, or the legal issues of business ownership, you're an expert in helping people heal.

In addition to fears around, "Can I do this?" our students also struggle with not being perfect at coaching and integrative nutrition and lifestyle medicine skills immediately. In the same way that you learned everything else in life, it will take time, practice, mentorship, and experience to be a great health coach with the ability to take an integrative clinical view with your clients. This will not happen overnight. Whenever this fear holds my students back, I ask them what it felt like to treat their very first patient as a licensed or certified healthcare professional. Did they do it perfectly? Were they super confident? In almost every case, the answer is no. They started shakily, learned through practice, and sought support and insights from their more experienced colleagues. The good news is that, once our students join The Women's Health Coach Certification, they become a lifetime member of our supportive community. We have students who graduated back in 2012 who still hop on our live coaching calls to get support with complex client questions or business challenges. We've always got your back!

A related fear is the fear of being criticized, especially by your peers. This is a challenge because it takes making yourself visible in order to bring awareness to your practice. As you share content, encouragement, and inspiration with your potential clients and community, you will make mistakes, and even when you do things well, it's always possible that someone will be there to criticize. During your training, we'll work with you to strengthen your boundaries, improve your ability to handle feedback (good or bad), and enhance your confidence so you can create better content, in writing or even on video.

Finally, our students struggle a lot with financial fears. They fear marketing and sales, get easily distracted by new shiny objects in the form of marketing tactics, and fear investing in their businesses before they are making significant money. While I am all for bootstrapping, you have to be willing to both hustle and invest. Building a business is a challenge – it's an extremely rewarding challenge, but a challenge nonetheless. To be successful, you must embrace the financial aspects of the practice. You must learn to enjoy the sales process and build your confidence around money and stay focused on revenue-generating marketing tactics, not just busywork.

THE INABILITY TO BE DECISIVE

To have a successful business, you'll need to develop your leadership skills. One of the most important capabilities of a leader is decisiveness. You won't always make the right decisions, and sometimes you'll have to refine your plan or scrap it completely and start over, but if you stay stuck, your practice will fail.

One of the most common decisions that our students struggle with making is to choose which ideal client they will focus on serving and what problem they will help them solve. Without commitment to an ideal client and key problem, all marketing tactics fail. When the marketplace can't tell who you're talking to, no one can hear you.

Lack of decisiveness is often a consequence of poor boundaries. When you say, "yes" too quickly out of a desire to please, or say, "no" too easily out of a fear of failure or exposure, you'll end up with a schedule that is not aligned with your goals. As Brendon Burchard famously said, "Email is nothing but an efficient organizing system for other people's priorities." When you avoid making decisions, it's difficult to chart your path, and even your daily schedule to reach the goals you (didn't) decide to set. Without clear goals and a clear strategy to reach those goals, you'll be easily distracted by the demands of others, shiny "opportunities" (that cost you time and money), and could even risk your business.

In fact, just recently, I was presented with two opportunities that looked great on their surface, a book deal and the opportunity to present videos of my content on a well-regarded web platform. But if I had agreed to the fine print on either of those contracts, I could have lost ownership of some of my core intellectual property. It was hard to give up two opportunities that looked good at face value, but I had to be decisive and turn them down to protect my ability to generate revenue from my content in other ways that I have more control over.

Fearing making a decision or letting others persuade us too easily are both recipes for your practice to fail. If your practice fails, you can't serve the clients who need you.

10

THE SECRET TO AVOIDING HEALER BURNOUT

As you transition your practice from a clinical mindset to a coaching mindset with an emphasis on improved autonomy and responsibility for your clients, this alone will reduce your burnout risk. But, like any other small business, a health coaching practice can be all-consuming. As the practice owner, you'll be responsible for the business itself, marketing, client care, and employee management. In short, you'll be responsible for everything. To make this easier on you and more effective for your clients, you must build a solid business foundation. Additionally, you must have clear boundaries about how you will run your practice.

A STRONG BUSINESS FOUNDATION WILL SET YOU FREE

All business involves taking risks. As clinicians, we tend to be risk-averse and focused on important details regarding scope of practice laws, client confidentiality, and our professional liability. This is important, but instead of letting fears around these professional issues hold you back, minimize that risk by putting appropriate accounting, legal, insurance, and financial processes in place. I am not a professional accountant, lawyer, insurance agent, or financial planner, so giving you advice in any of these professional service areas would be irresponsible. However, in our health coaching education and certification programs at The Integrative Women's Health Institute, we offer updated resources to support you in all of these areas. At a minimum, be sure that you have access to professionals to consult with in all of these key areas of business foundation.

THE COACHING AGREEMENT

The health coaching process requires a commitment from the client through a specific length of time to be successful. It's probable that, at some point, the behavior change work will get difficult, and your client may want to give up. The commitment is part of the incentive to overcome the barriers to change that have been getting in the way of her health for years. Thus, you and each of your clients must commit to a coaching agreement at the beginning of the engagement. This is distinct from clinical health-care, where once a person reaches their health goals, no matter how long it takes, you may be required to stop treatment, especially if that treatment is being paid for by a third-party payor.

Energetically, the coaching agreement signifies your commitment to each other as coach and client and the client's commitment to herself. Every coaching client must sign a coaching agreement before they commit to the process. This can be very powerful. We must be mindful not to abuse this power and only take on the number of clients that we have the bandwidth to give the required level of commitment to. This coaching agreement is a two-way street. Committing to only the clients you can serve with your available energy is an important decision you must make in your practice to practice at your highest level of ethics.

The coaching agreement is a legally binding agreement. You must create your agreement with the assistance of your attorney. Choose an attorney who specializes in health coaching and is familiar with the healthcare scope of practice laws in your state. You can practice more confidently when you have a clear agreement in place with your clients.

YOUR HEALTH COACHING PROGRAM CONTAINER

When determining what kind of business model (container for health transformation) to create, you must keep in mind the intersection between two things. First, what is your bandwidth and how do you like to practice? Second, what does your ideal client need to successfully reach her vision of health?

Consider the various health coaching models. You can build a practice that focuses on one-on-one coaching over time in person or via telehealth. You can build a group coaching program. You can build an online program that is augmented with health coach accountability support, and/or tracking and accountability with wearable tracking devices and apps. You can create in-person retreats or intensives with the time and space over an intensive period of time, such as a weekend or week for deep transformation. All of these models can work very well. But, as a business owner, in most cases, you can't run more than one of these models without burnout unless you have clear time boundaries and some support. Right out of the gate, avoid planning a retreat, building an online course, and starting a coaching program. Each of these services is a full business unto itself requiring marketing, sales, financing, management, customer service, and planning. In some cases, you can implement more than one of these business models over time, but that has to be done carefully with a lot of consideration.

Consider how you like to work. Do you like to really get to know your clients and spend time with them every week to support them to make progress over the long term? Or do you like the intensity of a shorter term, but focused transformative experience, such as a retreat? Do you like leading groups and facilitating that interaction? What kind of model for supporting your clients feels easiest to you? Which model capitalizes on your best energy flows? The more you optimize your service with your natural energetic rhythms, the easier it will be to maintain the energy to do this work. Coaching is not easy work. It requires intensity, focus, and mindful presence. It's not easier than clinical work, it's simply a different perspective. But it doesn't have to drain your energy if you set up your coaching container with deliberate consideration of how you do your best work.

Concurrently, consider what your clients need to be successful. Is their health challenge and vision deeply personal, such that it will benefit from one-on-one sessions over time? Or, will stepping into a like-minded community of healing support accelerate her healing? Would an intensive opportunity give her the space to step out of her routine and responsibilities and focus only on her health? There is no one right or wrong answer here. The better you get to know your ideal client, her challenges and needs, where she tends to get stuck, how long it takes for her to see results of her health behavior change, and the details of her vision, the better the container you create will become. This is another reason why it's so important not to commit to too many different services (or more than one ideal client) as you begin your coaching practice. Start with one service offering and commit to it for at least three years. With that level of commitment, you can iterate your service over time and with the experience of many ideal clients taking their coaching journeys inside of the container you created. Your experience along with that of your ideal clients will allow you to refine your service over time.

GET STARTED! HOW TO CREATE YOUR FIRST HEALTH COACHING PROGRAM

Based on eleven years of health coaching practice where I have tested many containers, I have found that, for my ideal clients with complex pelvic pain conditions, a four-month program combining an integrative approach to nutrition, lifestyle medicine, and the health coaching process is best for my ideal client population.

You'll start creating your first program offering by taking your best guess at the ideal container for your ideal client to reach her vision. Consider the following:

- What kind of assessment and/or self-assessment will she need at the beginning of the program to assess where she is now, compared with her vision and goals?
- How often will she need coaching sessions for support?
- Will it be easier for her to reach her goals with group support?

What other support resources might she need along her healing journey, including health resources such as surgeons, physical or occupational therapists, massage therapists, or fitness instructors, and including home resources such as childcare, cooking support, or friends to laugh with?

Will wearable fitness and health trackers or digital apps help to monitor progress, support accountability, and inspire goal achievement?

Will your client likely need any supportive educational materials, such as guided meditation audios, recipe guides, or checklists of natural skincare product options?

How long will it likely take for her to at least see measurable and noticeable progress toward her goals that will keep her motivated to continue?

When you create your first coaching program

container, consider it version 1.0 of your program. Over the next several months and years, you will keep improving your program as you receive feedback from your clients. You can't optimize your program by thinking about it alone in your office. You must take it out into the real world and use it. As the Reid Hoffman, co-founder of LinkedIn once said, "If you're not embarrassed by the first version of your product, you've launched too late." Don't wait to start working with people. Experience and feedback are what will make you a better clinician-coach, and feedback from your clients is what will make your program more effective for your ideal clients.

What about the price? I am often asked by my students how they should price their initial program offerings. Surprisingly, the answer is, it doesn't matter. When you're first starting out as a coach, you might not feel sure of the value of your services. Should it cost the same as a massage therapy or physical therapy session per hour? Should my hourly rate be the same as a gynecology visit or primary care visit? What if, by completing my program, a client solves her pain and no longer needs surgery – should my program cost the same as the surgery? The answer is, it doesn't matter. Eventually, you will intuitively land on the right price based on the value of your offering to your client. For example, if your client gets her health issue solved in four months and can now work (and wasn't able to before), the value of your service is very high because you've helped her regain her ability to work. Or, if your service helps her to restore her energy, providing her with the ability to be a more patient and present parent, what is that worth? As you gain experience with working with your ideal clients and seeing them get great value from your work together, you'll develop the confidence to value your program appropriately. In the meantime, use borrowed confidence and start with a program rate between $500 and $2000. Your client is not paying for an hour of your time but for the value of the result you will help her to achieve.

ENROLLING CLIENTS IN YOUR HEALTH COACHING PROGRAM

Ahhh…the dreaded sales and marketing section. I'm going to keep this simple. All marketing tactics work, but only if that tactic is utilized with your ideal client in mind. Would your ideal client use the social media platform where you're marketing or attend the event where you're speaking? When you create marketing content to share in social media posts, on stage at events, or anywhere else, are you speaking to your ideal client? If not, then none of the marketing tactics will work. The goal of all of your marketing tactics is to eventually invite your ideal client to a sales call.

Don't freak out, this isn't a slimy process. In fact, your sales call with a prospective client should be a coaching call. The goal is to give value to your potential client during this call and mutually determine if working together will be a good fit for both of you. Your "sales" call process is simple:

Step 1: Ask your client where she is now in her healing journey, where she would like to be (her vision), and why she is stuck getting between here and there.

Step 2: Mindfully listen to her answer for at least ten minutes without interrupting her, other than the occasional reflection or clarifying question so that you're sure you're understanding her, and she knows that you're listening with intention. This step alone is a healing gift to any potential clients who join a sales call with you.

Step 3: Decide if you think your program can help her move from where she is now to where she wants to be in terms of her health goals.

If you don't think your health coaching program can help her, let her know that and, if possible, offer her some resources that can help her. Ask if there is anything else you can do to support her at this time, and end the call.

If you believe your program can help her, move to Step 4.

Step 4: Tell her the basic information she'll need to know about your program and how you think it can help her to reach her goal. Ask her if she has any questions.

Step 5: Answer all of her questions.

Step 6: Invite her to make a decision about whether or not she would like to enroll in the program. If yes, have her enroll in the program.

Step 7: Orient her to the program. Let her know if she will receive anything from you. Discuss scheduling or any other necessary details. Orient her to her role in the process, and send her the coaching agreement and any other required paperwork to sign.

It's that simple. Congratulations on enrolling your first health coaching client!

11

YOUR HEALTH COACHING PRACTICE VISION

Imagine that it's a typical Wednesday morning. You have complete control over your schedule. You have the luxury of working and recovering to your own biorhythms. Earlier, you had planned out your schedule to optimize your energy through the month, not based on an antiquated, masculine, industrial revolution, nine-to-five weekday workday. Just because you're working with your biorhythms, doesn't mean you're not working hard. You're more productive than ever because you're working when you're naturally energized and have built in time for self-care, recovery, and even laziness and pleasure!

You know your ideal client very well, and you keep learning more about her. Your insight into her needs allows you to anticipate them, and use your coaching communication skills to support her to bring her own wisdom for healing to the surface.

Collaboratively, you support her vision with goals, and she takes the reins to implement daily action steps like making her morning smoothie, getting her weekly powerlifting in, and committing to her nightly bedtime routine. When that's not enough, she asks for help from her professional and home Webs of Support. She leans on her teams of support, gathers their advice, falls into their hugs, and drops off her kids with them for much needed respite. She is steadily gaining the energy she needs to be an even more productive member of her community because she's regaining her health, and now she can devote even more energy to solving her community's challenges with homelessness and taking on new projects at work. Her relationship with her husband is improving and they reconnected to their mutual love of nature. She has the energy again to take longer, higher, and more breathtaking hikes with him.

The ripple effect of your work is vast, but it's not entirely dependent on you doing everything. You've learned to leverage your services and receive payment for the value of your work. You've taken risks, put yourself out there, and become more decisive. This journey has not been easy, but as a member of the Integrative Women's Health Institute community, you've found that someone always has your back, that it's okay to be afraid sometimes, and that you're stronger than you think. You have learned that you don't have to know everything to start, that the experiences you gain from working with your clients and getting support from your community are the best teachers.

You used to be afraid of technology. You went into healthcare because you like to use your hands, not stare at a screen. But you've learned the power of technology to allow you to reach clients who live in rural towns or tiny apartments far beyond your hometown. You've learned that you can bring women together who feel alone and the community that you have created is part of the medicine you prescribe.

With the wisdom you have gained by reading this book, you can do this on your own, but it will be easier if you do it within our Integrative Women's Health Institute Community. By joining our health coach training programs, you will have the community and coaching you need to stay accountable to your own goals. Learning these skills of health coaching communication, functional nutrition and lifestyle medicine, and business, sales, and marketing will be a new challenge. Just like when you learned your clinical skills, you'll have questions, you'll be confused about how to prioritize your next steps, and sometimes you'll get stuck. That's perfectly normal. It's all part of the learning process.

Remember the day you saw your first patient in the clinic on your own. You probably felt a little nervous (or scared to death!), but then you remembered that you were trained for this. You spent years in school learning the skills to help the person sitting in front of you. Your transformation from clinician to coach will be the same, but better. There is no need to forget everything you've already learned and practiced. Now, you have the opportunity to utilize new skills, a new way of thinking, and a new way of supporting your clients. The key difference is that this coaching method of practice is not designed to burn you out. It's designed to care as much about your health as your client's health. Why healthcare wasn't designed in this way in the first place will always remain a mystery to me.

When you join our health coach training programs, we'll go beyond teaching you new skills. We'll coach you and surround you with a community that cares about your success and your health. Just last night on our Women's Health Coach group coaching call, we spent an hour discussing and coaching through sleep challenges. Not just for our clients, but for our coaching students themselves. It's a well-used refrain that we "can't pour from an empty cup." It's shocking that the current healthcare system does nothing to fill the cups of its healers.

This acute healthcare crisis has opened the door of opportunity to create a new model of health practice. Are you ready to walk through it? Are you ready to learn the new skills of a modern coaching model of healthcare practice? Are you ready to shift your perspective and let go of the controlling clinical mindset? Are you ready to prioritize your own health as an essential part of the healing work that you're doing? Are you ready to take risks and willing to receive the rewards that will open up to you when you risk being seen and being decisive?

If you're ready to transform from clinician to coach and be a leader of the healthcare transformation, join us! I can't wait to see what you create and the millions of lives that are healed because you were willing to step into your power.

ACKNOWLEDGMENTS

Thank you to every one of our Women's Health Coach Certification students and graduates. It's my privilege to witness the expansive coaching practices you create.

Thank you to all of the professional coaches I have learned from over the years, especially My Dad aka The Original Mike the Coach, Fabienne, Jordan and Steve, Angela, Tonya, and Greg.

Thank you to the many hands that made this possible, especially Nadja, Analia, Emily, Vari, Scott, and our amazing IWHI Master Coach team, Susan, Susie, Naja, Cathy, Liz, Amy, Angela, Cindy, and Melanie.

Thank you to my family. I couldn't think of a better team to quarantine with. I love you Mark, Claire, and Kate and can't wait to see what you continue to create in this world!

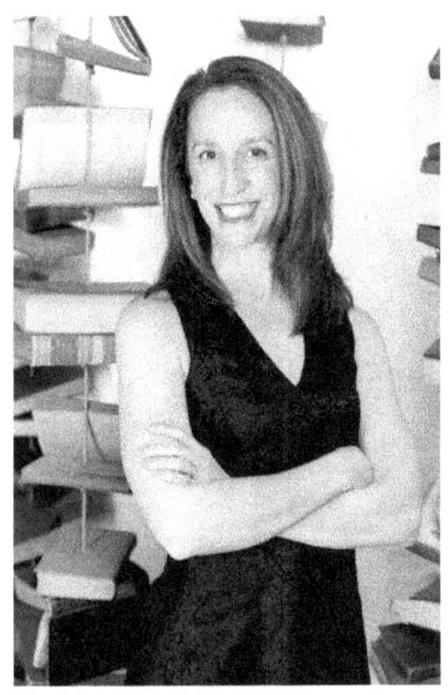

Dr. Jessica Drummond, DCN, CNS, PT, NBC-HWC is the founder and CEO of The Integrative Women's Health Institute and the bestselling author of *Outsmart Endometriosis* and *Clinician to Coach*. She is passionate about caring for and empowering people who struggle with women's and pelvic health concerns. She is equally passionate about educating and supporting clinicians and wellness professionals to confidently and safely use integrative tools to transform women's and pelvic healthcare.

Dr. Drummond has two decades of clinical experience as a licensed physical therapist, licensed clinical nutritionist, and board-certified health coach working with women with pelvic pain, including endometriosis, vulvodynia, and bladder pain syndrome. She brings a unique, conservative, and integrative approach to supporting women to overcome hormonal imbalances, and chronic pain conditions. She is a sought-after international speaker on topics such as integrative pelvic pain management, natural fertility options, optimal hormone health, menopause, and female athlete nutrition.

She loves farmers markets, art museums, eating great food, and having girls' movie nights with her daughters. She lives and works from her home and offices in Fairfield, Connecticut and Houston, Texas reaching thousands of clients and professional students in over sixty countries through her virtual practice and educational programs.

Dr. Drummond was educated at the University of Virginia, Emory University, Duke Integrative Medicine, and Maryland University of Integrative Health.

ABOUT DIFFERENCE PRESS

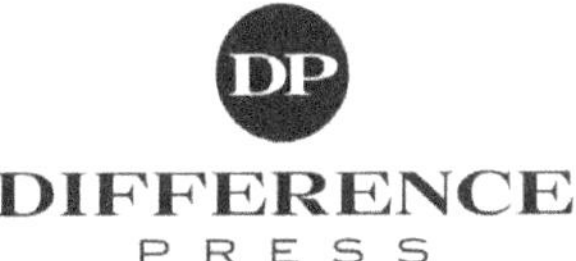

Difference Press is the exclusive publishing arm of The Author Incubator, an educational company for entrepreneurs – including life coaches, healers, consultants, and community leaders – looking for a comprehensive solution to get their books written, published, and promoted. Its founder, Dr. Angela Lauria, has been bringing to life the literary ventures of hundreds of authors-in-transformation since 1994.

A boutique-style self-publishing service for clients of The Author Incubator, Difference Press boasts a fair and easy-to-understand profit structure, low-priced author copies, and author-friendly contract terms. Most importantly, all of our #incubatedauthors maintain ownership of their copyright at all times.

LET'S START A MOVEMENT WITH YOUR MESSAGE

In a market where hundreds of thousands of books are published every year and are never heard from again, The Author Incubator is different. Not only do all Difference Press books reach Amazon bestseller status, but all of our authors are actively changing lives and making a difference.

Since launching in 2013, we've served over 500 authors who came to us with an idea for a book and were able to write it and get it self-published in less than 6 months. In addition, more than 100 of those books were picked up by traditional publishers and are now available in bookstores. We do this by selecting the highest quality and highest potential applicants for our future programs.

Our program doesn't only teach you how to write a book – our team of coaches, developmental editors, copy editors, art directors, and marketing experts incubate you from having a book idea to being a published, bestselling author, ensuring that the book you create can actually make a difference in the world. Then we give you the training you need to use your book to make the difference in the world, or to create a business out of serving your readers.

ARE YOU READY TO MAKE A DIFFERENCE?

You've seen other people make a difference with a book. Now it's your turn. If you are ready to stop watching and start taking massive action, go to http://theauthorincubator.com/apply/.

"Yes, I'm ready!"

OTHER BOOKS BY DIFFERENCE PRESS

The Successful Canna-preneur: The Practical Guide to Thrive in the Legal Cannabis Space by JM Balbuena

Healing the Healer Within: 8 Steps to Unleash Your Potential by Dr. Cheri McDonald

Ocean of Possibilities: Maximize Natural Cancer Healing with Marine Organisms and Functional Medicine by Heather Moretzsohn

Will I Ever Get Pregnant?: The Smart Woman's Guide to Get Pregnant Naturally Over 40 by Tsao-Lin E. Moy

The Evolving Home: The Conscious Design Guide to Restoring Function and Comfort in the New Normal by Kadie Remaklus

Voices of Fibro: The Guidebook for Moms Seeking to Care and Support Their Child Living with Fibromyalgia by Mildred Velez

Ultimate Fulfillment: A Blueprint for Finding and Living Your Purpose by Dr. Joy Kwakuyi

Thank you so much for reading this book. I hope you enjoyed learning about how simple it can be to transform your practice from a stressful clinical model to an expansive coaching model. I hope you feel more empowered and have a clearer plan for your career of service. The world needs you to step up and be a leader in this healthcare transformation.

As my gift to you, I'd like to give you some bonus materials to support this book.

To get access to these free materials, go to http://clinic2coach.com.

Let's connect!

You can follow updates, research, and inspiration on my website, and social media channels.

Website:
http://integrativewomenshealthinstitute.com/

Instagram: https://www.
instagram.com/integrativewomenshealth/
Facebook: https://www.
facebook.com/integrativepelvichealth
Twitter: https://twitter.com/jessrdrummond
LinkedIn: https://www.linkedin.
com/in/jessicarobilottodrummond/

www.ingramcontent.com/pod-product-compliance
Lightning Source LLC
Chambersburg PA
CBHW071622150726
48000CB00004B/1837